Praise for *Invisible Chains*

"I wish I'd had this book in my youth, when I was the victim of coercion that whittled away at my self-esteem. This book should be in every women's center, police station, and therapist's office. It cuts through the jargon, gets to the heart of the matter, and provides tools of liberation." —Magdalena Gómez,
author of *Shameless Woman*

"The first comprehensive guide to overcoming coercive control. Dr. Fontes provides simple tools to assess your own or a loved one's relationship and offers practical steps to getting free, illustrated with real-life stories. The writing is sharp and evocative and the research is impeccable. A pathbreaking work."
—Evan Stark, PhD, MSW, Professor Emeritus,
Rutgers University School of Public Affairs

"Dr. Fontes makes the dynamics of coercive control understandable to everyone. In plain language and with clear examples, she describes the tactics of domineering individuals and their effects on victims. Dr. Fontes is particularly thoughtful about including diverse couples and families. After reading this book, no one will be able to ask, 'Why does she stay?' "
—Juan Carlos Areán, Director, National Latin@ Network
for Healthy Families and Communities

"This book reveals hidden dimensions behind relationships where one partner is controlled by the other. Dr. Fontes explains the dynamics of coercive control and deciphers the pattern so we can all understand it. Read this book and reclaim your life." —Rabbi Efraim Eisen, marriage, family,
and child therapist, Amherst, Massachusetts

INVISIBLE CHAINS

Also by Lisa Aronson Fontes

For Professionals

Child Abuse and Culture:
Working with Diverse Families

Interviewing Clients across Cultures:
A Practitioner's Guide

invisible chains

Overcoming Coercive Control in Your Intimate Relationship

Lisa Aronson Fontes, PhD

THE GUILFORD PRESS
New York   London

Library of Congress Cataloging-in-Publication Data
Fontes, Lisa Aronson.
    Invisible chains : overcoming coercive control in your intimate
relationship / Lisa Aronson Fontes.
      pages cm
    Includes bibliographical references and index.
    ISBN 978-1-4625-2024-4 (paperback) — ISBN 978-1-4625-2035-0
(hardcover)
    1. Dominance (Psychology)   2. Control (Psychology)
3. Interpersonal relations.   4. Intimate partner violence.
5. Intimidation.   I. Title.
    BF632.5.F66 2015
    158.2′4—dc23

                                                          2014048835

For my children, Marlena, Gabriel, and Ana Lua,
with love and gratitude

Contents

Purchasers of this book can download and print a larger format of the
questionnaire on pages 127–136 from *www.guilford.com/fontes3-forms*.

About This Book

This book discusses relationships where one person dominates and intimidates another in an abusive process called *coercive control*. These relationships usually are not "all bad." Coercive control often feels like love. Passion and companionship can exist alongside threats, punishment, isolation, and even physical violence.

> Coercive control often feels like love.

Coercive control is a special kind of torment because it happens within a relationship of strong personal bonds, hopes, and dreams. Coercive control continues over a period of months, years, or decades—unlike a one-time assault by a stranger, for instance. Coercive control wears down a victim's autonomy and sense of well-being over time. Between the direct acts of control and possibly violence, a victim lives in fear. The distress is ongoing, even during periods that seem calmer.

Women can certainly be as bossy and jealous as men. However, for reasons discussed later, coercive control almost always involves a man using a range of tactics to hurt, threaten, degrade, and isolate his female partner. Coercive control does sometimes involve a woman as the oppressor and a man as the victim. It can occur in relationships involving gay, lesbian, bisexual, and transgender people as well. This book is designed to assist all people who are controlled by their partners, whatever their culture, age, gender, or sexual orientation.* Coercive control among LGBT[†] people, and in relationships where women dominate men, are the focus of Chapter 5.

This book includes both "everyday" and extreme examples. Some of the subtle forms of coercive control can be hard to detect and may feel like love when they first appear. For instance, a woman may feel flattered that her partner wants to be with her at all times: driving her to work, meeting her for lunch, and accompanying her when she shops. Family and friends may commend her for finding such an attentive mate. He insists he is motivated by love and concern for her safety, so she pushes aside the discomfort she feels about never having time alone. His frequent texts during the day sometimes interfere with her work. On several occasions he grows angry because she doesn't respond promptly to his calls or texts, or because she spends time with a friend without asking him first. Then he begins to check her cell phone and upsets her with his constant questions. While no one of these acts in itself appears overly alarming, they build up over time. The woman becomes less and less free.

In contrast to these "ordinary" acts, the more extreme examples included in this book are obvious signs of abusive control and may prompt readers to ask, "Why would anyone put up with that?" Chapter 4 explains the dynamics that keep women in relationships where they are controlled and victimized.

The examples in this book are all based on real situations, although I have changed identifying details to protect privacy. They are drawn from my work as a psychotherapist, community activist, workshop presenter, and researcher, as well as personal

---

*The pronouns ("he or she," "him or her") become quite complicated if used in every sentence. Most of this book uses pronouns that describe the more common situation of a man controlling a woman.

[†]The initials LGBT are used here to signify people who identify as lesbian, gay, bisexual, or transgender. The language we use evolves constantly. I hope those who identify as queer, asexual, pansexual, and so on, will be able to find themselves in these pages as well.

conversations in many settings. Some of the examples come from my own experience as a former victim of coercive control.

This book is divided into four broad parts. Part I describes coercive control, the ways it shows up in some couples, and how it affects victims. Part II seeks to explain why some people use coercive control against their partners, and why it is difficult to break free. Part III discusses coercive control of LGBT people, heterosexual men, and teenagers. Part IV offers strategies and advice for ending coercive control.

For easier reading, this book includes very few citations. Accessible and relevant readings and Web links to organizations are listed in the Resources at the back of the book.

HOW TO USE THIS BOOK

Use this book in whatever way works for you. Some people will want to thumb through it and take a look at the stories. Others will want to read this book quickly, over the course of a day or so, from beginning to end. Or you might prefer to start with whichever chapter seems most relevant to you and read a few pages each day. You could choose to keep notes separately or record your reactions to the book in the margins. If you are currently in a relationship that includes coercive control, make sure you keep your book and notes in a safe place so you will not be punished for having them. This book may trigger upsetting memories in people who have been physically, sexually, or emotionally victimized. Please take care of yourself as you read this book. Seek help from others or put the book down for a while if you feel "triggered" by some of the stories here.

WHO I AM AND WHY I WROTE THIS BOOK

I have a doctorate in counseling psychology and specialize in difficult family issues. I have been at turns a psychotherapist, researcher, professor, trainer, consultant, and activist in the areas of child abuse and violence against women for 25 years. In the course of my work, I have spoken with professionals and community members in settings ranging from a church in Ohio to a shantytown in Chile to a hospital in California. I have trained physicians in Massachusetts, police officers in Pennsylvania, military social workers in Germany and Texas, firefighters in New York, and psychologists, social workers, nurses, and advocates across the United States and Latin America. I have worked with parents, grandparents, and other caretakers in volunteer organizations, in psychotherapy, and in their own neighborhoods. I am the mother of three young adults.

I have also listened. I am no longer a practicing psychotherapist, but when I was, I listened to women and men of all backgrounds describe their relationships. I have had the privilege of conducting research and networking with people from all over the United States and the world—especially with people who speak English, Spanish, and Portuguese. I have worked with refugees. The books, articles, and chapters I have written are widely cited.

However, my greatest lesson in coercive control was deeply personal. After my 25-year marriage ended, I entered a relationship that became increasingly controlling over time. From those few harrowing years, I found out what it means to be subject to another person's whims. I experienced, directly, the fright of being stalked during the relationship and after ending it. Even with a high level of education, knowledge of violence against women, a steady job, and a strong network of friends and family, I felt utterly trapped. I grew to appreciate, firsthand, the dedicated professionals who help people survive and exit these relationships safely, and recover. My friends and family helped me regain my balance. I learned how very long it can take to recover, and I learned that recovery is possible.

Evan Stark's groundbreaking 2007 book, *Coercive Control*, helped me understand what had happened to me and to many women and a few men whom I have known over the years. I felt stronger as I learned names for the traps that had confined me. I began to see patterns where previously I had seen only separate, painful moments.

Stark's book is directed at scholars in the field, and has prompted a whirlwind of interest in coercive control. To help this important concept reach a broader audience, I have written this shorter, nonacademic book. I developed advice for people who are being victimized. I created sections on same-sex couples, teenagers, male victims, and people in the military. I coined the term "coercive entrapment" to describe the most extreme cases of coercive control.

I wrote this book to help people avoid being caught in a web of coercive control, improve those relationships that can be improved, and disconnect from those that are toxic and will not change. This book also aims to reach professionals and friends and family of people in controlling relationships, so they can understand and lend a hand to people who are being victimized. No one should have to struggle alone.

This book highlights the need to raise boys to become men who will treat one another—and the women in their lives—with kindness and respect, rather than violence and control. It shows why we should never be asked to give up our freedom and self-esteem to be part of a couple. In the interest of caring, supportive relationships, please read on.

PART I

What Is Coercive Control?

Criticism. Isolation. Threats. Sometimes even physical abuse. These are the weapons of coercive control, a strategy used against some people by their intimate partners. It usually includes some combination of degrading, isolating, micromanaging, manipulating, stalking, physically abusing, sexually coercing, threatening, or punishing. A relationship that should involve loving support ends up a trap designed for domination. Victims feel anxious, dependent, and afraid, deprived of their freedom, self-esteem, and basic rights.

Chapter 1 introduces coercive control. Chapter 2 describes its far-ranging tactics and their effects.

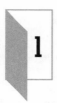

Introduction to Coercive Control

When 23-year-old Lily's boyfriend, Dave, started quizzing her about where she had been and she caught him examining her phone, she decided Dave was "a jerk" and broke up with him immediately. Dave texted her several times a day for a couple of weeks, and once she saw him sitting in his car outside her workplace. But that was the end of it.

Mandy, age 35, did not see her situation so clearly. After the whirlwind courtship in which Tom showered her with cards and flowers, Mandy married him. Then he started asking Mandy for details about how she had spent her day, with whom she had spoken and for how long. Tom complained about how much time Mandy talked on the phone with her mother and sister. They had their first real fight when Mandy arrived home with short hair, and Tom was angry that she had cut it without asking for his opinion. She promised to grow it long again. It seemed as if nothing she did pleased him. Over time, Mandy noticed fewer loving moments and felt increasingly anxious about Tom catching her doing "something wrong." With two children at home and feeling worse and worse about herself, Mandy felt trapped.

Lily and Mandy were not simply unlucky in love; they were victims of coercive control. Coercive control strips away victims' independence, sense of self, and basic rights, such as the right to make decisions about their own time, friends, and appearance.

Coercive control shows up in a variety of relationships. This book focuses on the most common situation: where a man uses coercive control against a woman who is his partner in an intimate relationship. Chapter 5 discusses coercive control in same-sex relationships and in heterosexual relationships where the woman dominates the man.

Many men who use coercive control also abuse their wives and girlfriends physically or sexually, sometimes causing severe or even fatal injuries. Others limit themselves to slapping, pushing, grabbing, and other types of force that might look mild to outsiders who don't see how frequently they occur and the fear they cause over time. Violence is one among many tactics of a strategy of coercive control. Some men use coercive control without physical violence.

Coercive control can sometimes be found outside romantic and sexual relationships. Coworkers and supervisors sometimes use coercive control at the workplace. And we find a similar dynamic in cults and other organizations, on sports teams, and in the military, especially during basic training. However, intimate relationships are especially ensnaring. The controller may have access to the victim around the clock and knows her daily routine. He may also know things about her that she has shared with no one else, such as her secret hopes and fears. She may have told him about experiences that she does not want to become public. He uses these secrets to control and hurt her.

Outsiders may not be able to see the signs of coercive control in a couple. The men who use it often make a good impression in other settings. Much of society still thinks men's control over women is just the way things are, and that what happens in couples is their private business. All this adds to a woman's sense of being imprisoned by her partner.

Coercive control is largely invisible.

Victims* of coercive control often feel like hostages. Over time, being grilled, criticized, and shamed may come to seem routine. Victims often blame themselves as they feel despairing and disoriented. It can be hard for them to figure out exactly what's wrong. Isolated and humiliated, some women lose confidence and accept their partner's view of reality. They may have trouble deciding whether their partners are doing and saying hurtful things out of love and concern—as claimed—or out of cruelty. They may feel confused as they are told again and again that they themselves have triggered their partner's behaviors by doing something wrong. At the same time, to keep the peace in their relationship, victims may detach from family and friends, contacting them less and less often until they lose touch with many of the people they care about most. Unfortunately, the victims typically do not see the connection between their partner's control and their own isolation until time has passed. Losing self-confidence and close relationships at the same time can be paralyzing.

> Victims of coercive control may be criticized, shamed, and punished regularly. They often feel like hostages.

Women who get caught in the web of a controlling man are no different from other women. They just had the bad luck to become involved romantically with a controlling person at a time when they were especially vulnerable. Once a controlling man has caught a woman in his web, he will do everything he can to prolong the relationship.

Victims of coercive control come from all racial, ethnic, and religious backgrounds. They live in mansions, trailer parks, city apartments, and suburban and rural homes. Often victims of coercive control keep up a happy front because they feel ashamed or because their partner demands it. Sometimes other people sense that something is wrong, but are not sure what. The woman may appear unusually shy, lonely, meek, or even disturbed. It may be

---

*I am using the word "victim" here to stress the power dynamic. Readers who prefer another word such as "survivor" should feel free to substitute it.

obvious to other people that she is being controlled, or the control may remain perfectly hidden.

People who exert control often look charming on the surface. To outsiders, they may even seem like ideal partners when they take over all crucial decisions. Some abusers appear eager to help others, friendly, romantic, and outgoing, while others seem mean and let their possessiveness show. There is no easy way to spot a person who will someday begin to exercise coercive control over his partner.

When he first meets a woman he likes, a controlling man will often say he wants to support and help her. He may buy her gifts, listen to her stories, and offer her advice about her work and family. He may do chores for her. He may look at her with admiration and think of her success as an extension of his own. If she is with a man like this, a woman initially benefits from his caring and concern. Family and friends may comment about the positive aspects of the relationship, saying, "You are so lucky to have found this man. You will never find another man like him!"

A part of her may feel uneasy, wondering, "What will happen if I don't want to follow his advice?" She is apt to brush aside these feelings because she welcomes so much of what he offers. She will avoid making waves. The abuser has communicated that it is better to just "go along" with his ideas and avoid conflict.

If a man acts romantic, charming, and supportive at the beginning of the relationship, his partner thinks this helpful man is the "real" him, and if she does things right, he'll go back to being helpful again. He may briefly return to his helpful self for a while, if this seems like the best way to maintain his control.

Over time, things usually worsen. Some controlling men start to see the woman's success as competition or as somehow making their own achievements seem less important. Others insist that outside activities of any kind distract her from meeting their needs and attending to housework and children. Many become jealous of all contact with others, even of the time a woman spends with her family. Life becomes what is called a "zero-sum game," in which whatever a woman gains in achievement, respect, or friendship is seen as taking away from her partner. The controlling man knows that if his partner grows and develops, she may refuse to put up with his restrictions. So he begins to stand in her way. His supportive advice turns into criticism. He acts like an expert on her life and career—as if he understands it better than she does. He views all of her outside involvements as signs of disloyalty.

A controlling man does not necessarily live with the woman he dominates. Sometimes he "dates" and controls her from a distance, by stalking her and disrupting her work and her relationships with friends and family. Because coercive control crosses so many spheres of a woman's life, simply "leaving" or ending the relationship may not end the problem. His abuse may continue or even escalate after the relationship is over.

A controlling man has many ways to impede a partner's progress. He blocks her access to the people and resources she needs to live her life on her own terms. He makes it inconvenient for her to study, discourages her from taking a promotion, or disrupts her work. He may interfere with her friendships and family ties, block her access to transportation, prevent her from learning new skills, and frustrate her attempts at self-improvement. Let's look at three brief examples of how coercive control can block a woman's advancement.

Jocelyn wanted to take college courses when her youngest child started kindergarten. Her husband, Jay, wouldn't hear of it, although this had been their plan when they married. He told her she needed to be available for their children in case one got sick during the school day. He discouraged her so strongly that she gave up her plans.

Christine decided she was drinking too much and wanted to give up alcohol. She told her husband, Ray, that she was going to stop drinking beer with dinner. Ray grew furious and accused Christine of trying to control him. On her first night without drinking, Ray refused to say a word during their meal. He accused her of behaving as if she was too good for him, and told her he hated to "drink alone." He offered "a compromise." She would drink with *him at dinner, but he would stop her when she drank too much. Christine gave in and drank with him—it just seemed easier. In this way, Ray pushed Christine to abandon a goal, and made sure that her head was clouded by alcohol, hindering her ability to think about her future.*

Teresa was a rising star in her city's painting world when she began to date Samuel, who also painted but earned his living waiting tables. Samuel was romantic but moody. Once, when angry, he threw a book at a wall. When he shouted at her, Teresa felt afraid. After a few months, Samuel moved his supplies into Teresa's studio space so he could work by her side. Samuel insisted they not paint on weekends, so they could devote themselves fully to each other. Teresa's painting suffered from Samuel's continuous presence and demands.

In couples where one person controls the other, the person who is being controlled cannot reach her full potential. Her partner stands in the way of her personal and professional growth. She not only feels trapped, but she also increasingly adopts his worldview as her own, losing her sense of who she is as a separate person.

> **A controlled person cannot reach her full potential.**

THE CONTINUUM OF COERCIVE CONTROL

No single act defines coercive control. A number of acts occur together, and a pattern develops over time. This book describes coercive control in general and provides numerous examples of specific acts. Certainly not all controlling men exhibit every behavior mentioned here in its worst form. One man cooks for the family but restricts his girlfriend's friendships and forbids her to hold a job because of his obsessive jealousy. Another man takes away his wife's paycheck and controls every cent of their finances but does not interfere with her friendships. One man rarely raises his voice but often threatens his girlfriend with physical harm if she does not do what he asks. Another insults his wife and keeps her from seeing friends and family but claims he would never hurt her physically. In coercive control, the abuser's moods, behaviors, and beliefs severely limit and alter his partner's. The overall concept of coercive control may describe a relationship even if not every example of bad behavior applies.

> **The concept of coercive control may describe a relationship even if not every example of bad behavior applies.**

On the other hand, not every man who is "bossy" is guilty of employing coercive control. There are many degrees of bossiness. But if the woman feels actual fear—if she feels she must respond to his demands *or else*—then she is probably a victim of coercive control. If she avoids saying and doing things that are important to her, for the sake of keeping the peace and avoiding conflict, then she is probably a victim of coercive control. In coercive control, the abuser uses threats, punishment, and criticism to limit his partner's access to resources such as friends, family, work, money, and freedom of movement.

Coercive control exists on a continuum.

Noncoercive (cooperative) relationships:
Mutual support and shared decision making. Arguments may surface. Neither partner frightens, threatens, or punishes the other. The couple balances connection and autonomy in a way that benefits both people.

Coercive control relationships:
One person uses a variety of tactics to control his partner. She buries some of her desires, plans, and opinions to avoid conflict and punishment. She may resist in hidden ways but grows increasingly isolated. She may experience physical and psychological symptoms.

Coercive entrapment:
Coercive control strategies are intensified by structural inequalities that further deprive victims of resources. The victim feels trapped, isolated, fearful, and threatened almost constantly. She may lose a sense of herself as an independent human being.

Not Coercive   Coercive Control   Coercive Entrapment

Is someone controlling you?

- Do you feel threatened?
- Are you afraid to speak up?
- Is your partner constantly jealous or possessive?
- Does your partner try to limit your contact with family or friends?
- Do you work hard to avoiding "provoking" a bad reaction in your partner?
- Do you feel ashamed of things your partner does to you or makes you do?

If the answer is "yes" to one or more of these questions, read on.

This book usually uses male pronouns to describe the controlling partner, and female pronouns to describe the person who is victimized, because these are the most common coercive control relationships. However, in no way should this book be seen as casting blame on all men. Most men do not control their female partners in the ways described in this book. Many men respect their partners and support their interests and work. Increasingly, men who live with their partners share housework and child care.

Men are also becoming involved in the fight against violence against women. Some do this formally, by joining antiviolence organizations, marching alongside women to "take back the night," and speaking out in their schools, workplaces, and communities. Other men do this informally, by telling friends, neighbors, workmates and even men they do not know to "knock it off," and stop being rude or unkind to women.

Readers may reject some of the terms used in this book, such as "controlling," "abuse," and "victim." Even the term "coercive control" may feel uncomfortable. The word "partner" is an awkward way to describe a wife, husband, boyfriend, girlfriend, or fiancé, but it's easier than providing that long list each time. Please do not get caught up in the terms. If you can relate to a situation but don't like the term, feel free to substitute another word that you think fits better. Most important here is to recognize when one person's pattern of behavior is making

> his partner feel afraid and humiliated with the consequence that she sets aside her own hopes and dreams just to get through the day without conflict.

People in same-sex coercive control relationships will find that almost all of the content here applies to their situations, even though many of the examples portray heterosexual couples.

Fortunately, it is possible for victims to break free of coercive control through their own actions, with the support of people who care. This book explains how to do it. The process builds on the steps that a victim is already taking to stay safe and limit the damage to her life and her self-esteem. As advocates, therapists, police officers, medical providers, clergy, and the legal community begin to understand coercive control, they will be better prepared to support the victims who need their help. They will also be ready to step in sooner and tell a controlling man that he must *stop* his abusive actions and respect his partner's humanity.

> Victims can break free of coercive control through their own actions. This book will show you how.

COERCIVE CONTROL IN CONTEXT

Not very long ago, other kinds of interpersonal abuse were finally recognized as social problems, named, and considered crimes for the first time. This is an important step toward eliminating them. For example, today we identify violence against a romantic or sexual partner as "domestic violence" or "intimate partner violence." We define sexual assault in intimate relationships as "acquaintance sexual assault," "date rape," or "marital rape." Stalking was described and made a crime, not only for Hollywood stars who are pursued by fans, but also for people who know each other. Recently, stalking laws have been extended to protect current and former intimate partners. Sexual harassment in schools and jobs oppressed women for centuries before people finally understood it, named it, and said, "Enough is enough." In 2014, sexual assault on college campuses and in the military gained new visibility.

Statutes and structures are finally being directed toward eliminating sexual assault in these institutions. We can see progress in combating those destructive forms of behavior. Now, at last, the time has come to shed light on *coercive control* in intimate relationships.

Those of us who work with victims of abuse in couples often hear that "the violence isn't the worst part." Attacks on self-esteem and independence can hurt as much as physical blows. These forms of social and psychological violence have recently been gathered together under the term "coercive control," one of the most common and devastating forms of abuse. Coercive control is usually supported by gender traditions that support men's power over their female partners.

Controlling another person is the foundation of all abusive relationships, including those that are physically violent. In many countries, including the United States, certain elements of coercive control are considered a crime. These include physical and sexual violence, criminal harassment, kidnapping, and stalking. Other behaviors—such as frequent telephone calls or showing up at a person's workplace—are not crimes by themselves, but they can be included in protection or restraining orders, which does criminalize them. In recent years many countries have broadened their definitions of partner abuse to include coercive control. For instance, in some European nations coercive control is considered a "course of conduct crime." This means that a series of harmful actions add up to a crime, even when a single incident of the same behavior is not illegal. In the United States, coercive control is not yet written into criminal codes, but this may soon change.

> **Controlling another person is at the root of all abusive relationships, including those that are physically violent.**

In couples where coercive control violates the victim's human rights such as freedom of movement, it should be considered a crime and should be handled by the police and the courts. In other couples, the control may be unkind and morally wrong, but it has not yet crossed a line where it would be considered a crime. Still, victims do need help and protection. Victims who become isolated are more likely to have their situations worsen. Concerned friends and family and social services can help end the victimization. They can help the victim understand her situation and provide her with material assistance to end the relationship, if she so chooses. It is also important for communities to change the norms around how men treat their wives and girlfriends, pressuring abusers to respect their partners' humanity.

2

Controlling Behaviors

If we look at each tactic of coercive control individually, it may simply look like a sign of a less-than-ideal relationship. When we view these tactics together, we see they form a pattern of domination with far-reaching effects. This chapter explores the strategies one person uses to coercively control an intimate partner: isolating, micromanaging, stalking, abusing physically and sexually, threatening, punishing, manipulating, degrading, belittling, and controlling a victim through her children.

ISOLATING

A controlling man feels threatened when his partner's life does not revolve entirely around his own. He tries to control her movements, achievements, and connections with others. Whether he is motivated by a sense of entitlement or insecurity or both, a controlling man deliberately tries to weaken his

> A controlling person feels threatened when his partner's life does not revolve entirely around his own.

partner by cutting off her access to resources such as meaningful relationships and money. This isolation and dependency force a woman to make the man's desires central to her life, while ignoring her own needs.

A controlling man serves as a filter for a woman's contacts with the outside world, gradually forcing her to lose the help and support of her family, friends, and coworkers. An isolated woman loses her sense of identity apart from the way her partner defines her. She loses avenues to express herself. After living this way for months or years, the woman may have trouble remembering how she once thought and felt and what she used to believe. As she has been deprived of meaningful contact with others and forced to take on the abuser's perspective, she may lose touch with her own values and preferences. After living like this for a while, an isolated woman may begin to lose the sense that she has a "self" to express. Being in a relationship of coercive control is like being in a cult. The victimizer gradually transforms the victim until she has lost touch with her former self. Like a cult leader, he isolates her, decides how they will live, and refuses to listen to others' opinions.

Cutting Off Contacts

A man may isolate his partner in many ways without appearing cruel or controlling. His efforts to have her all to himself may initially feel like love. He just cannot get enough of her. He says he wants to protect her from harm and doesn't want her to tire herself out. A controlling man often chooses a woman who is younger and less worldly and cloaks the ways he restricts her freedom in statements about keeping her safe. But this isolation does her serious harm.

A controlling man isolates his partner to make her dependent on him, express his ownership over her, monopolize her skills and resources, and keep her from getting help or support. He might move his girlfriend or wife to a home far from her family and friends, where she does not know people and is likely to feel lonely. He might limit her phone calls, insist that she share all her social media or e-mail contacts with him, and require that she talk to friends or family "on her own time," such as during the workday, so he can have her undivided attention in the evening and on weekends.

A controlling man often isolates a woman by making it difficult for her to be alone. He may insist on joining her in activities she previously enjoyed without him, such as grocery shopping, clothes shopping, or getting together with friends. Or he will insist she stop taking classes because he doesn't like her sitting next to male classmates. If he cannot accompany her somewhere, he may ask his mother or another family member to do so. Sometimes a controlling man provides far-fetched explanations as to why his partner should not engage in activities without him. For instance, if she has been in the habit of going running with friends, he may tell her she should stop this because running interferes with her ability to get pregnant. Or he may offer no explanation at all for why she should stop doing the things she enjoys, other than "Because I don't want you to."

Working outside the home does not protect a woman from coercive control, although it does enable her to avoid becoming completely isolated. Even while she's at work a controlling man can reach his wife or girlfriend through telephone calls or texts, computer messages, or dropping in unexpectedly. An abuser might obligate his partner to come right home after work and avoid socializing with coworkers. The bottom line for a woman subject to coercive control, regardless of whether she works outside the home, is this: she is unable to choose how and where she will relate to other people.

> People who work outside the home sometimes suffer from coercive control, but they are protected from becoming completely isolated.

Often women are closely connected to their families. For this reason, an abusive man might prohibit his partner from seeing family members. Or he might interfere in ways that make family visits short, tense, or infrequent. He might tell her it is time to transition from her role as a daughter to her new role with him, urging her to spend less time with her family. He might try to persuade his partner that her relatives are not good people, are a bad influence, or are harming their relationship. The abuser may listen in on phone calls, embarrass the woman in front of her family, intercept e-mails or social media, or destroy photographs, letters, and gifts. He might threaten or attack the woman's family.

A controlling man often tries to drive off his partner's support system. Behind her back, he might give her friends a negative picture of her. He knows just what to say to create conflict among others, without seeming to be doing this on purpose. He might threaten or intimidate her friends, or he might flirt with or even seduce one of them, or tell his partner that one of her friends flirted with him. He works hard to persuade his partner to reject people she has trusted in the past. His goal: to isolate her and make her more dependent on him.

Jack bought and poured generous portions of liquor for the friends of his girlfriend, Caitlin, when they visited and then told her she shouldn't hang around with those friends because they were drunks. Jack also talked to Caitlin's friends privately and told stories about her that he knew they wouldn't like, to push them away. Afterward, he told Caitlin that her friends had criticized her behind her back.

A man who uses coercive control often isolates his victims further by setting up tests of loyalty. The abuser defines any choice to spend time with others rather than alone with him as a sign of not caring. The abuser's "urgent needs" interfere with his partner's activities. For instance, at moments when his partner tries to stake out some time for herself, a controlling man might insist on having sex immediately, have a car accident, require an urgent trip to the doctor, or raise a scene that requires an extended conversation.

Abusive men commonly say, "What happens at home stays at home," claiming it is disloyal to speak with others about their life as a couple. While this may sound like a neutral statement pro-tecting the couple's privacy, such a statement makes it hard for the woman to seek outside support. It is part of an isolating strategy.

> Abusers commonly claim it is disloyal to speak with others about their life as a couple.

Cutting Off Access to Employment and Money

A controlling man often makes it difficult or impossible for his wife or girlfriend to work by demanding that she call in sick fre-quently or by embarrassing her at the workplace. Getting her fired will result in furthering her isolation. He might tell her that he can take care of her material needs and therefore she should quit her job or not look for one. Or he might push her to take a job working for him. He might press her to have children, or more children than she desires, and then try to convince her that the children need her at home. He might isolate her by giving her a long series of household tasks to complete to such a level of perfection that she does not have time to do anything else. A controlling man might require his wife or girlfriend to attend to his sick or elderly relatives. Certainly women sometimes make these kinds of life-changing decisions on their own or in conver-sation with their partners. In coercive control, these decisions are imposed by the man to control his partner, and the isolation is compounded by other practices that will be discussed here.

Meredith, 36, worked for an advertising agency, where she needed to keep up appearances. Joe grew increasingly jealous of the time she spent working. Sometimes he hid her laptop, telling her she needed "to relax." Often he'd demand sex in the morn-ing, when she was ready to go out the door, making her late to her job. On the morning of a particularly important presentation, Joe grew angry and threw a cup of coffee at Meredith, staining her best suit and forcing her to scramble to get dressed again. Meredith coped as well as she could. She bought another suit and left it at the office. She e-mailed copies of her presentations to herself, so she would not be stranded if Joe kept interfering. None of Meredith's coworkers had any idea of what she was going through, although a few noticed that she looked more stressed and distracted than she has previously.

An abusive man might isolate a woman by controlling her finances, denying payment for basic needs, or taking away her money through threats, trickery, violence, and outright theft. He might demand that she pay all their joint expenses including rent, food, and utilities. He might deny his wife a credit card or insist that all their cards be held jointly and then deliberately ruin her credit. While he makes large expenditures on his own, he requires that she justify even small expenses. He demands that she deposit her entire paycheck into their joint account and gives her little money from it. Often the rent or utilities are under the woman's name and her partner says he will take charge of the bills, but he does not pay them. If his spending throws the family into debt, she becomes responsible for balancing their accounts by avoiding spending money on the household, herself, or the children.

Sometimes a woman pays for her partner's schooling, car, or equipment for work. Although he swears he will pay her back, he does not. When an abuser thinks his partner is getting ready to leave, or after she has left, he may try to force the woman to stay or return by making sure she is broke and has a poor credit rating. Without money, a woman's isolation intensifies.

Sometimes a controlling man provides his partner with money and a lavish lifestyle she could never afford on her own. Submitting to his every desire becomes the price she has to pay for benefiting from his wealth. If she tries to leave, he might present her with a bill, telling her she owes him a lot of money.

Ruining Her Reputation and Relationships

Some abusers isolate and control their partner by ruining her reputation or threatening to do so. For instance, a high school boy might threaten to spread sexual rumors about a girl if she does not do what he asks. A woman who faces this kind of situation may react by withdrawing from social contacts, not sure whose opinion of her has been contaminated by her controlling partner or ex-partner. The stories he tells about her do not have to be true to cause damage.

It is not unusual for a controlling man to want to know very personal things about a woman as they begin to date. At first this might feel like a welcome sign of love. As time goes on, she sees that he can use his knowledge as a weapon to control her.

Coercively controlling men often show near-constant jealousy, making it difficult for their partners to attend ordinary social events or relate normally to others. A controlling man might accuse his partner of flirting or being involved sexually with friends or coworkers. Or he might tell her that another person is "hitting on" her and she just is not bright enough to notice.

> A person's extreme jealousy can make it hard for his partner to interact normally with others.

Women often report having to be extra careful about what they say and do, including how they dress and apply makeup, so as not to provoke their partner's jealousy.

In what may seem like a contradiction, sometimes a controlling man pushes his girlfriend to sexualize her interactions with others. He might do this because he feels sexual ownership over her. He might also grow sexually aroused by watching "his" woman excite someone else. He might harbor homoerotic feelings and enjoy watching another man's arousal, imagining that he is in his partner's shoes. As long as he is in charge of these contacts, he may believe he can avoid feeling jealous.

Bobby pushed his girlfriend, Mersayda, to wear tight, low-cut shirts when they went out, even to family events. When in public, he would ask her which of the men in the room she found most attractive, and he'd push her to flirt with them. He made her answer the door in lingerie when workmen showed up. Bobby scolded Mersayda if she refused to play his "games" but also criticized her if he thought she seemed to enjoy them too much. Mersayda often felt like hiding, ashamed of the way she had to present herself at Bobby's insistence.

An abuser distorts and strains his partner's relationships when he sexualizes them, whether through jealousy or through transforming neutral contacts into sexual ones.

Isolating through Technology

Controlling men commonly tamper with women's cell phones, interfere with their computers and infiltrate their electronic communications, as discussed in the section on stalking (pages 30–32).

> **Controlling people commonly tamper with their partners' cell phones.**

Increasingly, couples exchange numerous digital messages and photographs. A controlling man may use this virtual trail to ruin his partner or ex-partner's reputation. He might pressure his wife or girlfriend into taking intimate or sexy pictures, or he might take photos or videos without her consent. Then he threatens to send the pictures to her friends, family, coworkers, or bosses—to everyone on her e-mail, Facebook, or phone list—if she does not do what he wants. Entire websites and blogs now exist filled with what has been called "revenge porn," sexy photos and videos posted mostly by men to exact revenge on a former partner.

Peter spent at least an hour each day watching pornography, which his wife, April, did not enjoy. He pushed her to have sex with other men, to join a swingers' club, and to stay at a swingers' hotel with him. Although April sometimes accompanied Peter in watching pornography or going places where swingers gathered, to keep him happy, April could not bring herself to have sex with another man. When April moved out and told Peter she wanted a divorce, he replied that he held records and photographs from every place they had visited and would send them to her supervisor, mother, children, and others if she did not move back in.

At first, April felt helpless and frightened. Then she realized that she could create a much longer and more damaging list of the things Peter had done wrong, from prior arrests to immoral and illegal behavior and using his office computer for pornography. April confronted Peter with the list and told him she was no longer willing to put up with his bullying. She told him that if he ever assaulted her reputation, she would do the same to him. He backed off.

Sometimes abusers incite others to send a woman repeated mean messages. Using information technology to harm or harass another person in a deliberate, repeated, and hostile way is called "cyberharassment" and is a crime.

Sometimes controlling men pretend to be the woman in social media, which is a crime. These acts can destroy a woman's reputation and put her work and social life at risk.

Sam created an account in the name of his ex-wife, Sandy, on a popular shopping website. He posted strange comments and reviews of sex toys and pornographic books in her name. He also hacked into Sandy's e-mail account and sent slightly inappropriate messages to her clients, coworkers, and boss. These messages were just off-color enough to cause others to withdraw and cause her boss to call her to a meeting. Sandy explained what was going on to her boss. He expressed sympathy but also said he was terminating her contract because they didn't want to "have to deal with that mess" in the workplace. The boss encouraged Sandy to reapply when she "straightened things out."

Sam's actions are a form of identity theft and are illegal.

Cyberharassment comes in many additional forms and is a crime. Using text bombing, one person can send the same message hundreds of times from a computer to a woman's cell phone or send the same message to hundreds or thousands of people. State laws vary, but if the messages inspire fear, they may constitute the more serious crime of *cyberstalking*. (See the section on monitoring and stalking, pages 30–32, for additional information on cyberstalking.)

Isolating Immigrant Women*

Whether they are partnered with other immigrants or with men who are native to the country where they live, immigrant women often face unusual isolation. Perhaps they do not speak the language, share the customs, or look like the people around them. They are especially vulnerable if they come from traditional cultures that support men's dominance and women's subordination, frown on divorce, and shun women who defy their husbands. If counseling and services for abused women do not exist in a woman's native country, she is less apt to use them in her new land.

Abusers may exaggerate the dangers of their new country to keep women locked fearfully inside. One professional man from the United States moved his Japanese immigrant wife and child to the suburbs and then told her she was too absent-minded to learn to drive. Dependent on him to go anywhere, she had no opportunity to learn English or make friends. In London, a Caribbean man refused to buy his wife clothing suitable for the city's harsh winters, making it nearly impossible for her to leave the house for months in her sandals and cotton dresses.

Women who do not have proper immigration documents are particularly vulnerable to abuse. Controlling men take away their wives' legal documents, avoid helping them become legal

---

*In the United States, people who are victims or witnesses of domestic violence, sexual assault, trafficking or other crimes may be eligible for the U visa, T visa, or the VAWA self-petition program, any of which may help them gain citizenship. Information is available online and from agencies that work with victims of violence. (See the Resources section in this book.)

residents, and threaten them with deportation if they try to speak up for themselves. Often controlling men lie to their partners about their eligibility for citizenship.

The Special Isolation of Military Families

The isolation of military dependents in many ways resembles that of immigrant women. Military families regularly settle into new housing, where at first they know no one. Families are on different move cycles at bases and in post neighborhoods. As one family comes in, a neighbor may have only six months before moving on. The dependent, usually the wife, may become fast friends with a neighbor only to have that neighbor move away in a short time, leaving her without a support system once again.

Moving frequently stresses military children's friendships and schooling. Because the family is one of the few stable features of their children's lives, a military wife and mother might decide to keep trying for family harmony rather than separate from her abuser. This can come at great personal cost.

The military sends families all over the world. Officers are usually moved every three or four years; enlisted people may move more often. The military member will be living apart from his family for long periods while he is away on assignments. Friends outside the military often do not understand the lifestyle and also may be in different times zones, making it difficult to connect at a distance. Therefore, the dependent is apt to find herself increasingly alone.

When a military member leaves for temporary duty assignments or deployments, his wife learns to function without his help. Whatever her role before his absence, she must take care of daily household responsibilities herself. If they have children, she makes decisions alone about their care, schooling, and discipline. She and the children get into a routine. Although she may be exhausted, she often gains confidence as she successfully guides her family on her own.

After his tour of duty, the military member is coming back to a family that has changed. Children have learned to turn to their mother for advice, not to him. His wife has learned to make and trust her own decisions. The family may even have thrived without him. If he is insecure, he may resent that he is no longer needed in the same way. To compensate, he either withdraws or punishes his wife for her new strength. He might try to remind his family who "wears the pants" by becoming a bit of a dictator.

The military member is used to working in a situation where orders are given and followed, and disobedience deserves punishment. He may try to apply these ways of interacting to his partner and children, who are apt to resent being treated as underlings. Being accustomed to a rigid hierarchy with a clear sense of right and wrong may make the complex interactions of family life frustrating. Because of their military training, some men become arrogant and lose their ability to reflect on their own behavior or to show empathy for others.

Military spouses and children are expected to be well behaved and to sacrifice for the country by supporting the service member. The entire community in and around a military base revolves around the soldiers and sees them as heroes. It is easy for the wife to blame herself for any relationship problems. After all, he has shown courage and loyalty to the country and to his fellow warriors—how could he be at fault? She is also likely to have heard, often, "Stay strong! You are a soldier's wife." In this context, "stay strong" means that she should put up with the difficulties that come her way, in support of her man and country.

If a military dependent is subject to control or abuse by her partner, she might be hesitant to speak with people in other military families, for fear of hurting her husband's reputation and career. Military families often decline to take advantage of the various forms of counseling available to them, for fear of hurting the service member's career and thereby putting their income, housing, and retirement plan at risk. A spouse who is being controlled or abused by a military member often feels utterly alone.

Counseling and domestic violence resources in the community and outside the military are apt to provide her with important sources of support.

Coercive Entrapment

If extreme isolation is combined with some of the other tactics outlined in this book, a person might be controlled to such an extent that we would describe her as being a victim of *coercive entrapment*. A victim of coercive entrapment becomes focused on surviving her immediate situation. She is consumed with trying to figure out how to act better and be more pleasing, in a continuing effort to satisfy her partner and escape his punishments. She may grow despairing and disoriented. Some controlling men deliberately weaken their partners physically, waking them repeatedly at night, restricting their access to food and medical care, obligating multiple unwanted pregnancies, and beating or sexually assaulting them.

> A woman who is exceedingly isolated and controlled may be a victim of *coercive entrapment*.

Cara had to "earn the privilege" of leaving the house by performing sexual acts for her husband that she found repulsive and painful.

Marla's husband locked her in their apartment each morning and unlocked her when he returned home from work each evening, saying it was for her own protection. He took her to the grocery store, as a reward, if he felt she had "been good."

Gita's husband would not let her go anywhere unaccompanied. He insisted on sitting in on her medical appointments, explaining to the clinic staff that this was "cultural."

Over a period of years, Hattie's boyfriend had whittled away at her health and her self-esteem to the extent that she hated to have anyone look at her—she could barely stand to see herself in the mirror.

Coercive entrapment may include crimes such as kidnapping or criminal confinement. The abuser's behavior is especially unnerving because it is so unpredictable. Women in situations of criminal entrapment feel desperate and hopeless. Sometimes they fight back or lash out against their abuser, hoping to save themselves from annihilation.

Resisting Isolation

People do not easily give up their right to make decisions about their own lives, including seeing friends. A woman who is isolated through coercive control looks for ways to connect safely with others. She strikes up conversations in places of worship, at the beauty salon, grocery store, or her children's school. She may schedule regular visits or phone calls with

> A person who is isolated through coercive control looks for ways to connect safely with others.

friends or family, and join a gym, book club, or parents' organization. She may seek out others on the Internet, get a job, or go back to school. She may keep money hidden somewhere, for her own use or to pay for her children's needs. A controlling man thwarts these efforts by prohibiting them and making them inconvenient or impossible. He goes to great lengths to discover how his partner is connecting with others and hassles her until she stops. A woman who is controlled coercively learns, over time, that her partner will make it difficult for her to interact meaningfully with others. Nevertheless, connecting with others is key to her long-term well-being (see "Resisting Every Day," pages 91–93).

MICROMANAGING EVERYDAY LIFE AND SETTING RULES

A controlling man asserts his dominance by setting rules and micromanaging his wife or girlfriend's everyday life. He might restrict her food and activities. He might insist that she take medications that he believes will make her thinner, more docile, or more interested in sex. A controlling man might govern how his partner expresses her emotions, what she watches on television, and which sites she visits on the Internet. Each day, he might decide what clothes she will wear and require rituals related to hygiene, exercise, or beauty. Implied in each one of the demands is the assertion "If you do not do what I say, I will punish you." Women follow the rules because to oppose them openly would raise uncomfortable or dangerous conflict. Complying with these rules reduces conflict in the short term but contributes to a victim's long-term isolation.

> A controlling person asserts power by setting rules and micromanaging his partner's everyday life.

A controlling man often exerts his control in spheres that pertain to a woman's typical gender roles. For instance, he might make elaborate demands regarding keeping house, preparing food, personal appearance, child care, and sex. He might demand that she be ready to receive, feed, and entertain his friends or colleagues at a moment's notice. An abuser might obsessively require that his partner put spices or canned goods in alphabetical order, iron his socks and underwear, fold towels in a certain way, or attend to household chores on an inflexible schedule, even when she is ill. This extreme behavior is different from a situation where the man is simply rigid and overly particular. In coercive control, the abuser's expectations become demands that his partner must fulfill with little regard to her own preferences or well-being, and she faces consequences for disappointing him.

A controlling man often institutes rules that cause his partner to live in fear of making mistakes. The rules might be so general that they are impossible to obey, such as "Never make me angry," "Always serve food that I like," or "Know what I want without my having to tell you." Sometimes the rules contradict each other, so a woman follows one rule while knowing she is going to "get it" for not following another. Typically, the rules become increasingly petty, so

> Rigid rules cause a victim to live in fear of making mistakes.

that infractions are almost inevitable. When a woman tries to explain why she has not complied with a demand or followed a rule, she may be told not to argue and to stop making excuses. Her partner keeps changing the rules, keeping her off balance.

Sometimes the rules appear to apply to both members of the couple, but serve only the interests of the abuser.

When they got married, Hector proposed a vow of "We will always put each other first." Hector would then remind Ashley of the rule whenever she tried to do something for herself. If Ashley pointed out that Hector had behaved selfishly, he dismissed her concerns.

One common rule is "sex on demand." The controlling man requires that his partner make herself available for sex when, where, and how he wants it. This requirement may be expressed explicitly, as in "I'm getting sex from you every day, whether you like it or not, so you may as well cooperate." Or, through a single instance of forcible rape, the abuser makes clear that "no" is not an option. The woman learns that saying "no" to sex would set her up for hours or days of hostility and is just not worth it. She learns to use sex to please her mate, to calm him down, and sometimes to help him fall asleep, so that he will leave her alone.

> One common rule is "sex on demand."

During the six months when they were dating, Violet and Lance spent every other weekend together while her children were with their father. They had sex at least once a day. Violet had not been in an intimate relationship since her marriage ended two years earlier, and enjoyed feeling physically connected to Lance and appreciated by him.

Lance insisted on moving into the small apartment Violet shared with her five-year-old daughter and six-year-old son. Lance demanded sex every night. He insisted that she have an orgasm each time. She began faking orgasms. She found it difficult to truly relax, especially since her children were in the next room. Once, when Violet said "no" to sex at night, Lance just sighed and rolled over, saying, "Okay." However, the next day, Lance began to ask her about why she was losing interest in sex with him. That night, he was rougher than usual when they had sex, leaving bruises on her arms. Violet quickly learned it was safer and easier to go along with Lance's sexual demands.

More information on coerced and forced sex can be found in the section "Degrading through Sex" (pages 51–54).

STALKING AND MONITORING

Stalking consists of a series of behaviors directed at a specific person, designed to make that person feel fear. While we commonly think of stalking as the way a crazed fan follows a movie star, stalking occurs most often within intimate relationships. And all too often, stalking continues or even worsens after the relationship ends. (See the section "If He Stalks You," pages 173–176, for more information on stalking after a relationship ends.)

> Stalking consists of a series of behaviors directed at a specific person, designed to make that person feel fear. Stalking can occur while a relationship is ongoing or after it is over.

A controlling man commonly monitors his wife or girlfriend's whereabouts, computer, electronic communications, mail, diaries, and phone calls. He might search her telephone, purse, pockets, closets, drawers, and car. He might also keep track of her time and money. He might obligate her to "check in" regularly by telephone, text, or photographs from her cell phone. He might ask the woman to chart what she is doing every 15 minutes or tell her what she needs to be doing every hour. Sometimes a victim of stalking in a relationship is not permitted even to close the door while she uses the bathroom.

A woman might feel obligated to stay at home all day, knowing her husband sometimes calls or stops by the house unexpectedly and would grow angry if he did not find her there.

Controlling men will often text or call their wives or girlfriends multiple times throughout the day and expect an immediate response.

Some controlling men try to convince their wives or girl-friends that they are watching them at all times. And—with the help of modern technology—this may be true.

Marta's husband, Sid, installed a GPS device in her cell phone that tracked her whereabouts. He also set up a program enabling him to see on his computer the phone numbers of everyone who called their home phone and the length of time they conversed. Marta suspected that Sid was reading her e-mails and confronted him. Sid tearfully confessed that he had been reading all her e-mails. He asked about e-mails that had troubled him, and she explained these for him reassuringly. He promised never to read her e-mails again and made a big show of uninstalling the spyware program. This was just an act; he continued to read her messages. In fact, he had installed a keystroke logger, a sophisticated program that tracked not just her e-mails but every key that she touched on her computer. He obtained her passwords and was able to read every e-mail, the text of every chat, and every post she made on social media.

Keeping track of another person in this way requires a lot of effort, time, and sometimes money. Some men invest hours each day in trailing their wives or girlfriends and following their foot-steps on the Internet.

A controlling man might obligate his partner to keep a log of her daily activities and interrogate her about any that could involve outside contacts, to the point that it's just "easier" for her to stay at home and live a diminished life. Sometimes these isolat-ing and controlling maneuvers are framed as good intentions, as in "I want you to write down everything you do during the day so I can help you make better use of your time."

Ordinary tasks and interactions come to feel risky to a per-son monitored in this way. A victim constantly wonders, "Will he disapprove? Could he misinterpret this? How will I explain this?

Could something happen that would bother him?" Being monitored closely leads some people to grow anxious and become afraid of situations that previously had never frightened them.

Some forms of monitoring constitute stalking and are illegal, especially if they form an intimidating pattern. Being stalked feels like wearing invisible handcuffs, tying a victim to her stalker at all times.

> **Being monitored closely leads some people to grow anxious and easily frightened.**

ABUSING PHYSICALLY AND SEXUALLY

Sometimes women are not certain whether the harm they are experiencing should be classified as physical abuse. A man who uses coercive control might engage in frequent physical intimidation that does not leave bruises. He might back her into a corner, grab her by the hair, hold her by the wrist, throw objects, or wrap his hands around her neck without squeezing tight. She feels threatened, but she may not see herself as a victim of violence. These are all violent acts, whether or not they leave a bruise.

What is the relationship between physical violence and coercive control? Physical violence is one possible tool of coercive control. Not all relationships of coercive control have physical violence. And not all couples with physical violence have coercive control. If a controlled woman has been harmed physically, outsiders are apt to view her as a victim, especially if they see bruises. But the damage done by the nonphysical control might be even greater.

Violence in couples is not always the same. These distinctions are important. Some couples fight physically when they argue. Either member of the couple may start the physical clash. Men usually inflict greater injury in these fights because of their larger size and experience with fighting. This kind of fighting has been called "couple fights."[1] This violence is often fueled by alcohol and by anger. The fights rarely result in severe physical injury

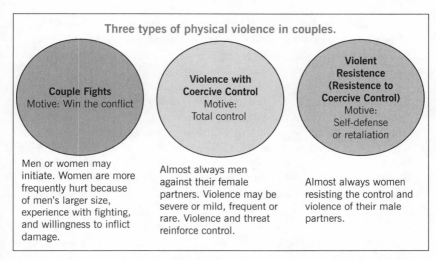

Three types of physical violence in couples.

Couple Fights
Motive: Win the conflict

Violence with Coercive Control
Motive:
Total control

Violent Resistence (Resistence to Coercive Control)
Motive:
Self-defense
or retaliation

Men or women may initiate. Women are more frequently hurt because of men's larger size, experience with fighting, and willingness to inflict damage.

Almost always men against their female partners. Violence may be severe or mild, frequent or rare. Violence and threat reinforce control.

Almost always women resisting the control and violence of their male partners.

(although accidents can happen), and they do not include the everyday domination of coercive control. This kind of violence in couples usually lessens over time. Police and other professionals who think they are hearing about or seeing evidence of a "couple fight" need to ask the right questions of each person, separately, to find out whether what they are seeing truly is a couple fight or whether coercive control is involved (see "For Professionals in the Field," pages 194–198).

In a second group of couples, a man who coercively controls a woman also abuses her physically and often sexually. In a couple where violence and coercive control both exist, the abuser's violence is motivated mainly by his wish to dominate. His acts of violence are intended to push his partner to change her behavior.

A person who uses coercive control may become violent as a part of his domineering strategy.

When Carl and Danette were in their first year of living together, Danette told him she was not happy and wanted to end their relationship. Danette said Carl's face changed and he slapped her so hard that she was afraid he had damaged her eye. Carl then apologized, brought Danette an ice pack, and kissed her. After this event, he threw away their condoms and insisted on sex. Danette complied. Carl began watching over Danette more carefully and restricting her movements. They had three children together. Carl never hurt Danette physically again in a dramatic way, although he occasionally grabbed or pushed her. Nevertheless, Danette understood that she was in a violent relationship throughout their years together. The control and threat of violence remained and shaped Danette's life every day. She feared that Carl might become even more violent if she tried again to leave.

Some coercively controlling men rely on constant low levels of violence—slapping, grabbing, pulling, and pushing their partners regularly. A controlling man might push his partner out of bed in the morning, slam the door in her face in the afternoon, elbow her at dinner if he doesn't like something she says, and have sex with her roughly at night. Some abusers are violent when sober, while others wait until they are drunk or high.

Fighting back against violent coercive control is termed "violent resistance,"[2] and this is the third kind of violence in couples. In the middle of an assault, a victim of violent coercive control might scratch, bite, kick, or pick up a weapon to defend herself. Or she might strike out when she feels backed into a corner. If some change in her abuser's behavior has led her to feel she or a loved one is at extreme risk, she might even kill him. Women who have been coercively entrapped sometimes end up killing their abusers.

Physical violence in couples can make it harder for outsiders to see the nonphysical control existing alongside the violence. The police, courts, therapists, and even friends, family, and neighbors may notice the visible effects of the blows but ignore other kinds of control. If the police become involved, legal charges are apt to be based on the physical assaults and not on the overall picture of control.

When police assess a violent domestic situation, it is important for them to understand and ask about coercive control as well as violence. Sometimes both members of a couple are arrested (or just the woman is arrested) when police are called to a home and see a man with scratches on his face, complaining that his wife "just went nuts." If the police were to separate the two members of the couple for questioning, they might discover that the woman's husband tracked her every movement, kept her virtual prisoner, and had been holding her by her neck at the time she scratched him.

If a woman uses violent resistance to escape from the control and abuse—for instance, by shooting her abusive husband while he sleeps—she may be judged entirely responsible for the shooting because she was not facing a physical threat at the very moment she attacked him. Her attack does not meet narrow criteria for self-defense. Throughout the Western world, attorneys, legislators, and advocates are working to change these unfair laws regarding violence in couples. Too many laws ignore the pressures of constant low-level violence, as well as continuous threats, isolation, and stalking.

Nonphysical forms of violence can damage victims' bodies as well as their minds. Living with chronic fear induces physical changes. Women who are victims of coercive control frequently experience medical problems, including heart trouble, headaches, and difficulties with sleeping and eating. It is fair to say, therefore, that all forms of coercive control have a physical side. In addition, all forms of physical violence affect a woman's emotions and her ability to think clearly.

Physical violence and coercive control reinforce each other. Even minor acts of physical violence make it easier to control a partner and intensify the effects of insults and threats. Similarly, people who feel entrapped and isolated become more afraid of physical blows. Once a woman is firmly under her partner's control, he may be able to keep her in check with occasional slaps and pushes, and he can refrain from more severe forms of physical violence.

The line between violence and safety can be especially blurry during sex. If a man leans too hard on a woman's arms or thrusts himself into her too brusquely and causes pain or spanks her in a way she does not like, she may be uncertain whether this qualifies as violence. If she asked him not to do these things and he still does them, she is a victim of violence. (This differs from a situation where a woman enjoys or requests submissive/dominant play during sex. If it is consensual, she is freely able to say "no" and he will stop, without pressuring her to continue.) If a man insists on sexual activities that a woman has said she does not want, or he handles her sexually in a way she has said she does not want, or he gets her drunk or high so she will do things she does not want, he is victimizing her sexually. Often, a woman gives her partner the benefit of the doubt if the painful actions occur during sex. She may decide to define his actions as passion rather than violence. In this way, the woman enables the relationship to continue without a risky confrontation. (For more information on sexual violence and coercion, see the section "Degrading through Sex," pages 51–54, and "sex on demand," pages 29–30.)

> The line between violence and safety can be especially blurry during sex.

Threatening and Punishing

A coercively controlling man sometimes threatens and punishes his partner to control her behavior. Threats and punishment have no role in healthy couple relationships. The threat implies, "Do this, or else," and the punishment provides a consequence for displeasing the abuser.

> Healthy relationships contain no threats or punishments.

Sometimes threats are open. An abusive man might threaten to hurt or kill his partner, people she cares about, or her pets. He might make suicidal gestures and threaten to kill himself. Suicidal threats show a victim the abuser's capacity for extreme violence. A controlling man might threaten to destroy a woman's reputation, have her committed to a mental institution, make her lose her job, steal her money, or destroy her possessions.

Often the threats are expressed physically rather than through words. An abuser might punch walls, slam doors, stomp around, and kick pets, to make those around him comply with his wishes or retreat in fear. Grabbing a telephone from a woman's hands or a child out of her arms are also clear threats. Even if these actions do not involve bodily harm, they create a climate of fear.

A controlling man might drive dangerously, with or without passengers, to intimidate his partner. He might tear up mail, slash tires or furniture, remove needed parts from a car, break windows, or throw away a woman's birth control pills. He might leave signs that only she knows are meant as a threat, such as putting the belt he has used to beat her on the dining room table or texting her a photograph showing that he is following her. Overturning a table full of food, spilling drinks, smashing dishes, and blocking a person's exit from a room are all forms of intimidation. Here is one extreme example of a man destroying property to intimidate his wife into staying with him.

With the help of a couple therapist, Debby asked Edgar to move out temporarily so they could reassess their relationship. Edgar agreed but told Debby on their way home from the session that she was going to be sorry. He packed one suitcase and moved to his mother's house that night. When Debby returned home from work the following day, her driveway was littered with broken glass. As she walked into the house with their two young children, Debby saw that the faucets were open, the sinks and bathtubs stopped up, and there was water everywhere. Debby felt unable to manage the flooded mess on her own and ended up calling Edgar. He cleaned up the glass and coached Debby in how to lie to the insurance company so they would be reimbursed for the flooding. Debby knew that lying to the insurance company was a *crime, but she felt like she had no choice if she didn't want to lose their investment in the house. Once she lied, Edgar threatened to expose her, saying, "I'll tell the authorities and then we'll both end up in jail. I don't care." Frightened, Debby broke off their couple therapy and submitted to Edgar for years afterward. Sometimes she felt like she wanted to die.*

In some cases, when a man stops taking needed psychiatric medication or stops going to an alcohol or drug treatment program, the woman knows he is doing this to intimidate her. Stopping treatment is his announcement, "Soon I will be out of control."

Abusers use punishments in coercive control in much the same way they use threats. Often an abuser will try to make a punishment correspond to the way he feels his partner has wronged him. So, for instance, if he feels his partner spends too much time talking to others, he might take away her phone, slap her in the mouth, or make her stay in the house all weekend. If she has burned the food, he might hold her hand over a hot flame. If he thinks she has nagged him too often about picking up his stuff, he might deliberately make more of a mess. Other controlling techniques discussed in this book, such as physical abuse and the silent treatment, can be used as punishments (see pages 32–36 and 42–44).

Guns and Other Weapons

Men who exert coercive control sometimes use weapons to threaten or punish their partners. The most common weapons are, naturally, extensions of the abuser's own body—his hands, his fists, his knees or feet, or his sexual organ, in a sexual assault. Many abusive men grab whatever object is closest—a belt, knife, wooden spoon, beer bottle, phone charger, or hammer, for instance. Some have weapons they use exclusively for threatening and/or punishing their partners, such as a whip or paddle. Some threaten their partners verbally with a vehicle—by threatening to "run them down," push them out of a moving car, or run them off the road. Others use the vehicle itself as a threat, by pinning a woman against a wall with a car, for instance, or driving up to her quickly before coming to a screeching halt and then laughing at her fearful response.

The weapons people use to threaten and harm their intimate partners vary somewhat according to where they live and their cultural background. People in rural areas often have access to hunting guns as well as farm imple- ments, cattle prods, and poisons. People in urban areas may be more likely to have access to handguns

> **Guns in the home increase the risk that someone will be shot.**

and switchblades. A farm worker may be more likely to threaten a woman with a machete, while a business executive may be more likely to swing a computer charger. In South Asia, some abusive men throw acid or boiling oil on women or pour gasoline on them and then set them on fire.

In the United States, the relatively easy access to firearms makes threats with guns quite common. A controlling man might threaten his partner, people she cares about, or a pet. Or he might shoot a gun into the air to show his lethal intention. Sometimes, the threats are less open but still clear.

Charlene knew that her husband, David, kept several guns for hunting and protection. Charlene had no doubt that David would kill her if he felt sufficiently provoked—especially if she attempted to leave. David did not assault Charlene. But when they were experiencing conflict, sometimes David would form the shape of a gun with his thumb and forefinger in a casual way. Charlene experienced David's hand gesture as a threat, and it immediately silenced her every time. He also cleaned his guns when he wanted to intimidate her.

Having guns in the home increases the risk that someone in the family will be shot.

MANIPULATING

Manipulating refers to the way one person changes another person's views or behavior through sneaky or deceptive means. Manipulation exerts a hidden power over another person. This serves the interests of the manipulator, often at the other person's expense. It is, therefore, a form of exploitation. When a person manipulates his partner, rather than simply asking for what he wants directly, he deprives her of the opportunity to make a free choice in response. This section explores lying, mind games, withholding, and using special skills and status to gain power

> **Manipulation exerts a hidden power over another person.**

over one's partner—all forms of manipulation.

Lying

Lying and telling partial truths strengthen a strategy of coercive control. Sometimes controlling men lie out of insecurity—to make themselves seem more accomplished in a variety of ways than they actually are. They lie to frighten their partners: bragging about their physical strength, their gang connections, or their past history of violence. Or they lie to minimize their problem-filled past, including drinking and drugs, womanizing, spending, gambling, and fighting. To create a certain image, they lie about previous relationships, their childhoods, and their jobs. They hide their controlling intentions and deny their actions. They spread false rumors to create rifts between women and their friends and families.

A person can manipulate his partner by rationalizing his own unkind actions, refusing to answer questions, or offering explanations that don't make sense. Often an abuser will blame the victim for his own actions. For instance, a boyfriend who has tried and failed to stop drinking alcohol will blame his girlfriend for his drinking, or a husband who has sexually abused a child will say his wife was at fault because she did not satisfy him sexually.

Sometimes controlling men create elaborate lies to cover up double lives.

Aldo was 82 years old when he met and charmed 70-year-old Samantha at a party. She had been divorced for 30 years and was delighted to be in love again, finally. They married rather hastily, not wanting to waste any time at their age; and then Aldo suggested they move from the large house she owned into a "more manageable" apartment, purchased with her money. Three years into this relationship, Samantha felt an envelope in Aldo's pants pocket while she was doing the laundry. It was addressed to a Aldo with a different last name and had been sent to a post office box in their town. Researching on the Internet, Samantha discovered that her husband had a different last name and another life in Italy—a wife of more than 50 years, children, and grandchildren. She finally understood that his long trips to Italy were not simply visits to his siblings. Samantha consulted a lawyer and the police as she planned her escape. Aldo had been so two-faced that Samantha was not sure what he might be capable of doing. She realized she did not know him at all, despite their years together. By the time Samantha got away from the relationship, she had lost a big chunk of her life's savings, which had consisted of the equity in her house. After their breakup Samantha learned that Aldo had charmed and married other women, whom he similarly fleeced and manipulated.

This interpersonal fraud is criminal. It is also a form of coercive control because it involves using an intimate relationship to deprive a person of her money and the ability to make decisions based on full information.

Women who are victimized in a controlling relationship may also lie. Sometimes they lie because their partners have demanded that they do so. For example, an abuser might instruct his wife to tell her parents that she does not feel well and therefore cannot see them. Most often, women who are victimized lie to protect themselves from physical or emotional abuse. These motivations are quite different from those of their abusive partners.

Withholding and the Silent Treatment

An abuser sometimes controls his partner by failing to behave in the way that would ordinarily be expected. For instance, a controlling man might refuse to listen, talk, or respond to his partner for long periods of time. This is sometimes called the "silent treatment." He may refuse to speak with her or even acknowledge her existence for hours, days, or weeks on end. Keeping silent serves as punishment, making a woman feel as if she is somehow less than human—like a ghost. Ignoring another person is not the absence of communication—it is a strong communication of power.

> The silent treatment makes a woman feel like a ghost.

Zaraiva could never tell what would set off her husband, Juan, and make him refuse to speak with her. Zaraiva first experienced Juan's silence when they were dating in Mexico. Juan felt that Zaraiva had looked too happy while dancing with her male cousin, so he walked out of the dance without saying good-bye. The two had been calling and seeing each other almost daily. For a week after the dance, Juan refused to answer when Zaraiva telephoned. Finally Zaraiva showed up at Juan's house, where his parents pushed him to speak with her. They went on a walk together. Juan responded coldly as Zaraiva wept. Juan eventually told Zaraiva that if she was "serious" about their relationship, he did not want her dancing with anyone else. He also told her that he was sick of "just fooling around" and wanted her to prove her commitment to him by having intercourse. Although she was a virgin, Zaraiva agreed. Soon she was pregnant.

   Over the years, Zaraiva learned to cope with Juan's cruel silences, continuing to prepare his meals and wash and fold his clothes even as he ignored her for hours, days, or weeks. The silent periods usually ended with Juan grabbing at Zaraiva brusquely for sex at night. The next morning, he acted as if the break in their relationship had never happened and refused to discuss it.

Being ignored is especially difficult for a woman who is iso-lated by coercive control and depends on the abuser's approval to feel valuable and safe. Many women would rather endure insults or shouts than the silent treatment. When they are shouted at, at least they know what is on the abuser's mind; and they feel better able to assess their own and their children's safety. Faced with stone-cold silence, women often feel desperately powerless.

Refusing to do chores or refusing to go to work *as a punish-ment* is a form of control through withholding. Withholding infor-mation can also be controlling (see the section on lying, pages 40–41).

Wendy was shocked one day to discover that her husband, Claude, had failed to pay the mortgage for several months and their house was going to be foreclosed. Claude had neglected to tell her that he was using their payments for gambling and had taken out loans in both of their names by forging her signature. (This is a crime.)

Another example of withholding important information is a person not telling his partner that he is involved in illegal activity that puts her at risk, for instance by storing street drugs in their home or car. Or an abuser might make a large purchase such as an automobile, boat, motorcycle, or even a house without telling his partner.

Some men withhold affection as a form of punishment.

Peggy's husband, Kirk, had insisted on sex almost every night in the two years since they were married. The sex seemed to be a way to help him fall asleep more than an act of love, and Peggy did not always enjoy it. However, when Kirk was angry he would not touch her. Instead, he masturbated in front of her each night and pushed her away if she tried to touch him. Kirk intended his no-touching and no-sex periods as a punishment. Peggy felt frightened when Kirk distanced himself physically. She knew it was a sign of his intense anger, which might explode in other ways.

Sometimes a controlling partner disappears without notice or explanation. He may simply fail to show up for dinner one night or fail to pick up the children as planned, spinning the household into worried chaos. Typically, when he does show up again, a day, week, or month later, he acts as if nothing has happened and criticizes the woman for being upset about his absence. Other men walk out the door in the middle of arguments, giving no notice about where they are going and when they will be back.

Of course, in many couples, there are times when one person does not feel like talking, doing chores, or having sex when the other does. But there's a difference when coercive control is involved. First, the act of withholding is more severe. Second, the withholding is part of a general pattern of control. Third, and most important, the motive for withholding is to threaten or punish the partner.

Mind Games and Gaslighting

Some abusers try to make their partners doubt their own memory, perception, or sanity. This has come to be called "gaslighting," after the 1944 film *Gaslight,* in which a husband deliberately tries to make his wife think she is crazy by dimming and brightening the gas lights and then denying that this is happening. He also isolates her by convincing her that she is too sick to socialize with others, and he hides objects and then convinces her that she was the one who had misplaced them. An abuser who gaslights his partner is trying to disorient her and make her seem crazy to herself and others, strengthening his control over her.

Mind games can range from small tricks such as turning the stove back on after a woman has turned it off to more elaborate manipulations.

Justin hid his wife's keys and purse and then would make them reappear. He would also remove some of her medication and tell her she had taken too much. Sometimes he moved furniture when she was out, or hid her cell phone, while denying that he had done

these things. Justin complained to friends that his wife was losing her mind. More important, he led his wife to doubt her own
perceptions.

Sometimes a controlling man uses technology to make a
woman doubt her sanity.

Sandra's boyfriend, Greg, had secretly installed a form of spyware
on her computer that allowed him to see every e-mail that she
sent or received. Occasionally, Greg used a phrase in conversation that she recognized from an e-mail she had sent or received,
and she found this uncanny. One day Sandra e-mailed her sister
about the "sweet and intense" life she shared with Greg. Hours
later, Greg commented in passing on their "sweet and intense"
life together. When she asked Greg about this coincidence, he put
his arms around her and said that he knew her so well he could
read her mind. She knew this was impossible, but she couldn't
help feeling that he could actually read her thoughts. From then
on, she tried to keep her thoughts "clean" while she was in his
presence. Sandra told a friend that she felt as if Greg had "placed
a computer chip in her brain." Sandra felt intimately invaded but
did not realize that Greg's "special power" was being achieved
through monitoring her computer.

A controlling man often acts charming, loving, and caring
when in the presence of others. When alone with his partner,
however, he may behave in blatantly cruel ways. This contrast
confuses the victim. She may hesitate to tell others about how he
acts when alone with her, convinced they will not believe her. She
may also have trouble trusting her own perceptions.

A controlling man sometimes intimidates his partner in
public by saying or doing things that only she knows are threats.
These acts can look like love to others.

Shavonda's boyfriend, Trey, would say something that included
the phrase "when we get home" when they were together in
public. By his tone of voice, Shavonda knew this meant he was
going to beat her. He would also have her sit on his lap when

with friends or family. This looked to others like an affectionate gesture. But while she sat on his lap, Trey would pinch Shavonda or whisper insults in her ear, all the while looking to others like a loving man. He would not let her move off his lap until he was ready. Inside, she was seething and unhappy. From the outside, they looked like an unusually affectionate couple. Shavonda kept up appearances because she felt it was her duty.

Manipulating through Status and Special Skills

Some people manipulate their partners through their position or area of expertise. For instance, an attorney who controls or abuses his partner understands both the law and the way it is enforced locally. He knows what he can get away with without having to face prosecution.

Similarly, the qualities that make police officers skilled in their jobs can also make them particularly successful at torment-ing women under their control. For example, officers have training and experience in intimidation, interro-gation, and surveillance. Officers also benefit from relationships with other officers, access to weap-ons, and knowledge of the law. A police officer who exerts coer-cive control over his partner often convinces her that it is futile to look to others for help. He uses his tremendous authority and close professional connections to keep her in line.

> Some people use thier job or status to control their partners.

Fields where a person holds authority over his partner are particularly ripe for exploitation. Some men use their workplaces to troll for girlfriends they can dominate. A divorce lawyer, for example, might take advantage of his female clients who are in crisis, using a client sexually and economically until he tires and moves on to the next victim. An art teacher might sexually exploit his students, persuading one after the other that he has chosen her as a muse and taking advantage of her trust and eagerness for his approval. A high-ranking administrator in a hospital might serially "date" women who work under him and then find rea-sons to terminate their contracts when the relationship ends. We often hear stories of music producers, agents, or sports coaches who sponsor and become the romantic partners of young women, demanding total obedience. A dog trainer might use his classes to find girlfriends and then use techniques of behavioral control with them. Gang leaders, military commanders, theater directors, supervisors, and bosses use their positions to control and sexually exploit their subordinates. The problem here is not that people occasionally meet each other through work, but rather that one person uses his professional power and authority over another and deliberately leads the more vulnerable person into a highly imbalanced relationship. These relationships are ripe for coercive control.

Frank, a psychiatrist, married Jenna, a social work student whom he met while she was doing an internship at the agency he directed. Jenna admired Frank's status and wisdom. Frank pushed Jenna to talk about her feelings. After the birth of their second child, Frank prescribed amphetamines (uppers) because he wanted Jenna to lose weight. The pills helped Jenna slim down and gave her the energy to handle their two young children. But Jenna became dependent on the drugs and soon was taking sleeping pills to "bring her down" at night. Although the medication had been his idea, Frank ridiculed Jenna for being dependent on the drugs and made her go without them for a couple of agonizing days, from time to time, saying she "needed to prove she could handle them." His true intention was to make her feel needy and unbalanced.

Jenna was increasingly confused during the day and often tried to catch up on the sleep she missed at night by napping. Then Frank complained about the condition of the house and accused her of being a bad mother. He lectured Jenna about her problems and belittled her opinions. Frank often "adjusted" Jenna's medication, telling her he was helping her resolve her "depression" or "anxiety." Frank ignored Jenna's complaints of side effects from the medications. Jenna had never suffered from mental health problems in the past, but over time she felt as if she was losing her mind. She felt less and less capable of running her own life. Frank's actions were unethical. Jenna gradually began to feel that she was "nothing" without her husband.

A number of cosmetic surgeons have "taken over" the appearance of their partners, molding them through procedures and surgeries, as if the women were experimental canvases. Controlling tattoo artists have been known to do something similar—tattooing, branding, and piercing women who have fallen into their web. If the person being marked in this way is a fully consenting adult, then this is her decision. However, sometimes the body modifications are part of a larger controlling strategy and take advantage of a woman's self-hate, timidity, or lack of self-esteem.

Ramona was just 17 when she walked into 28-year-old Tyler's studio for her first tattoo. Within six months she was covered in tattoos and piercings and had begun spending all her time at the studio, answering the phone and handling the appointment schedule. Ramona slept on one of the tattoo tables at night. She dropped out of high school just months before graduating. She tried the drugs Tyler and his friends gave her. Ramona felt as if she had entered into a secret and entrancing world. She liked being desired by Tyler, who initiated a sexual relationship with her (despite going home to his wife and children each night). Tyler "worked on" Ramona almost every day, piercing her lips, cheeks, eyebrows, and nipples and installing textured metal under her skin so that one arm looked as if it had scales. Essentially, Tyler did everything to her teen body that he could, in a short space of time.

Ramona allowed Tyler to hang hooks in her flesh and suspend her—for the intense experience. Tyler explained that suspension was part of a lifestyle, he was her mentor, and she would get better at it over time if she learned to "turn her brain off."

Ramona became almost unrecognizable to her family and friends during those rare times when they saw her. She was different not simply because of the changes in her appearance, but also because she was glum, edgy, nasty, and high much of the time. One evening Ramona's mother showed up at the tattoo studio after hours with her siblings. They persuaded Ramona to come home. The mother left a note telling Tyler she would press charges against him if he contacted her daughter again. Ramona entered into intensive psychotherapy to understand what had happened to her. Tyler had used his position to shape and control a vulnerable young woman.

Many professions have explicit ethical guidelines that pro-hibit intimate relationships with employees, students, patients, interns, or clients. Often these ethical guidelines are weakly enforced. Other professions do not have guidelines, or the guide-lines are unclear. Sexual harassment can easily slip into coer-cive control if there is an ongoing relationship. People who try to understand the control one person has over another should examine whether the controller's profession, skills, or status give him special ways to manipulate his victim. Some victims have difficulty getting help because their abusive partner's profession gives him extra clout in a "he says/she says" situation.

If the controlling partner is a therapist, an attorney, a doctor, or a police officer, a victim may have trouble turning for help to other people in her abuser's profession. Sometimes the victim can over-come this obstacle by going outside her geographic community, meeting with professionals in another town. Or she can seek help from a nearby domestic violence agency. An advocate at the agency might help her find professionals who understand the issue and the need for confidentiality. Or other kinds of resources might help her. For instance, if a woman is abused by her psychotherapist hus-band and would not trust other therapists, she might turn to peer support groups, or self-help materials available on the Internet.

BELITTLING AND DEGRADING

Belittling and degrading involve treating someone as an infe-rior—as a child or as not fully human. Many men who use coer-cive control deliberately belittle or degrade their partners to establish their "ownership" and moral superiority, and to dam-age the woman's self-respect. The controlling man feels better by making the woman feel worse. He feels powerful by making her feel powerless. He feels justified in abusing her because, in his mind, she is unworthy of better treatment. If he feels generally inadequate or in

> A controlling person often feels stronger when he makes his partner feel powerless and ashamed.

some way inferior to his partner, he may degrade her to bring her down and to "even things out."

More Than Just Insults

In many couples, insults fly back and forth or one partner might simply be rude; this does not mean they are in a relationship of coercive control. The belittling in a relationship of coercive control is one-sided and is more extreme or more constant. Victims report being told that they are worse than garbage, that no loves them, that their presence makes people feel sick, and that they are lucky the abuser is willing to tolerate them. In addition to saying mean things, the abuser deprives his partner of the social network that otherwise would help her feel better about herself. She is more fragile in response to his insults, because she is so alone. She does not feel that she can simply walk away from the insults; if she did so, he might act even worse.

> In coercive control, the insulting is one-sided and extreme or constant.

In a relationship of coercive control, the abuser's physical and social needs seem central at all times, whereas his partner's needs are minimized, denied, pushed aside, or distorted. He sets the terms, and she is expected to follow. He claims the right to make the large and small decisions. He decides when subjects are closed for discussion. If she does make small decisions—purchasing a small item for the home, for instance—he is apt to ridicule her choice. He may deliberately give her gifts she does not want and then blame her for not appreciating them. He makes plans without consulting her and then criticizes her if she objects.

An abuser tries to convince his victim that he knows what she needs better than she does herself. The end result: she is not able to make decisions about her own life.

Craig repeatedly told his wife, Ruth, that she was "always too busy" and "needed to learn how to relax." He obligated Ruth to sit by his side and "just be" for increasingly long periods of time, while he read or surfed the Internet on his computer. After ending the relationship, Ruth reported that she had felt like a dog being made to "stay." She said she was trained to accept Craig's instructions over time, after being convinced that he had her interests in mind and knew what was best for her.

Sometimes an abuser targets his insults toward his partner's areas of strength. If she is proud of her appearance, he will attack her looks. If she is proud of her cooking, he will not only criticize her cooking but also make sure he comes home for dinner late, so the food will be overcooked and he can blame her for it. On the other hand, some controlling men choose to attack their partners' insecurities. If a woman feels fat, for example, he might call her a "fat cow." If she feels insecure intellectually, he might constantly call her "stupid."

Controlling men often make women debase themselves in public.

Arthur insisted that his wife, Rosie, keep her gaze cast down when in public. He ordered her food at restaurants and answered for her in conversations. Arthur also insisted that Rosie walk in front of him when on the sidewalk, so he could watch how others interacted with her.

Degradation exhausts the victim and weakens her ability to resist. A woman often cannot respond to these restrictions and insults without putting herself at further risk.

Degrading through Sex

Many controlling men find ways to use sex to degrade their partners. Physically forcing a person to engage in sexual acts that she does not want is degrading—and is against the law in every state in the United States and most countries in the world, even if the two people are married. Many women find it extremely difficult emotionally to prosecute their husband—or even an ex-husband or ex-boyfriend—for sexual assault. Reporting the crime itself can feel humiliating, depending on how the criminal justice system handles it.

Sexual coercion occurs along a continuum. There is no coercion in acts that are decided on by both partners, together and freely. There is some coercion in acts that one partner agrees to reluctantly. A controlling man often pushes his partner to engage in particular sexual acts by letting her know she would face hassles or specific consequences if she refused. Victims describe coerced sex as among the most common and awful aspects of coercive control relationships. Using physical force to obtain sex is on the far end of the sexual coercion continuum. Physically forced sex is a sign that the relationship may turn lethal (see the Lethality assessment on page 138). A woman who has been physically forced to have sex once may feel this threat in the future, so that coerced sex becomes routine.

> **Coerced sex is humiliating and extremely common in coercive control relationships.**

Degrading sexual acts do not always involve physical force; they may range from actions that seem mild to various forms of

---

Sexual coercion exists on a continuum.

Not Coercive:	**Coercive:**	**Forced:**
Sexual acts that both members of a couple agree to freely and without pressure	Sexual acts under pressure, such as when one partner initially expresses reluctance or refuses but is then "talked into it," or when one partner consents to "keep the peace"	Sexual acts without consent, including rape and acts where one partner cannot give consent due to being drunk, drugged, or unconscious

←————— Not Coercive   Coercive   Forced —————→

torture. On the milder end, a man may pressure his wife to wear revealing clothes in public that make her feel uncomfortable. While this may not sound extreme, a woman in this situation is not being permitted to present herself to the world in the way she wants. This interferes with the way others perceive her and even with the way she sees herself. This is a form of public humiliation. Or a man might deliberately refuse to bathe before sex, as a way to assert his power over his partner.

In more extreme but quite common situations, the abuser pushes his partner into sexual acts that she finds painful or humiliating. Abusive men frequently use anal sex as a punishment, because it can be painful. He might penetrate her with objects or obligate her to engage in sexual acts with other men, women, children, or animals. An abuser might use unwanted sex acts as a punishment, using his penis or fingers as a weapon and her body as a target. He might deliberately pass on a sexually transmitted infection. An abusive man might force his partner to have sex in places where they can be seen by others or take sexual photographs or videos of her and then use these as blackmail to control her behavior. He might have sex with other women or men and obligate her to watch. A controlling man often rejects his partner's sexual overtures but then insists that she comply whenever he asks and in the ways he wants. If she declines to have sex with him or refuses to have it in a particular way, he might call her names, threaten to have sex with other adults or with her children, or simply rape her. He might obligate her to submit to painful and humiliating sexual "inspections," saying he is checking to see whether she has been aroused or sexually active with another man.

What do all the behaviors described in this section have in common? They deprive a person of the opportunity to decide when and how to express herself sexually. This is different from encouraging one's partner to be more adventurous sexually. This overture becomes coercive control if the abuser implies, "If you do not do what I want, I will make things unpleasant for you." When sex is used to degrade another person, it is all about the dominant person's desire for control. Degrading his partner and forcing her into acts she tries to reject gives some men an extra thrill. Others may simply believe they have the right to do whatever they want sexually with their partner or ex-partner.

Extreme Degradation

Some men degrade women through controlling their bodily functions such as toileting, sleeping, eating, drinking water, and even moving. Some men weigh their wives or girlfriends daily and control what they eat, oblige them to adopt peculiar or restrictive diets, or force them to take laxatives or submit to enemas. Others smear food or semen on the women's hair, deny their victims permission to use the bathroom, deny them toilet paper, or force them to eat food that has spoiled. Controlling men sometimes convince their wives and girlfriends that they are unattractive and persuade them to undergo cosmetic surgery such as breast implants to correct those "imperfections."

While some controlling men obligate women to exercise, follow diets, and/or wear clothing that is supposed to make them more attractive, others try to diminish their wives or girlfriends by making them less attractive:

Charlie let his wife shower only once a week and taunted her as smelly and disgusting between showers.

Doug punished his wife, Abby, by making her wear the same sweatpants and sweatshirt for weeks on end without washing them. As their relationship deteriorated, Doug began piling Abby's plate with food and would not let her leave the table until she had finished her meal. Then he called her "a fat pig" and told her that no one could ever love her.

More than once when he was drunk, Rodrigo took scissors to his wife's hair and deliberately left her with an ugly, lopsided haircut. When Rodrigo thought his wife had spoken too long with a male neighbor, he shaved off her eyebrows to "teach her a lesson."

Some men will bite, bruise, burn, cut, or tattoo their wives or girlfriends as a way of proving their ownership and inducing self-hate in the women. A violent man might also break or knock out a woman's teeth or scar her face. These practices are so common that the National Coalition Against Domestic Violence has established joint programs with the American Academy of Facial Plastic and Reconstructive Surgery and the American Academy of Cosmetic Dentistry to enable battered women and their children to have injuries and missing teeth repaired, and tattoos and scars removed.

In some extreme situations, controlling men treat women like animals by forcing them to eat out of a dog bowl or eat dog food, by forcing them to wear dog collars or tying them up, by making them go days without speaking, by using commands such as "heel" with them, and by refusing to allow them to sit on chairs or sleep in a bed, obligating the women to sit and lie on the floor. These extreme forms of degradation are alarming and indicate increased risk. It is important to remember, however, the milder but more common humiliations that make life tough for other victims of coercive control.

CONTROLLING A WOMAN THROUGH HER CHILDREN

Whether he is the biological father, stepfather, or simply the mother's boyfriend, a controlling man poses a risk to the well-being of any children in the couple's life. If he uses physical violence, he might directly assault the child, emotionally or physically injure the child while assaulting the mother in the child's presence, or

> Where there is violence in a couple, children suffer trauma, fear, and uncertainty.

even obligate the child to hurt his or her mother. Controlling men sometimes make a mother harm her own children. All too commonly, children—and especially boys—step in to defend their mothers, and suffer physical injury themselves. Where there is violence in a couple, children suffer trauma, fear, and uncertainty.

Even without physical violence, when a controlling man deprives a mother of the resources she needs to protect and provide for her child properly, he is placing her children at risk. For instance, her children suffer if he denies her access to education, transportation, or a job.

Distancing a Mother from Her Children

Connecting with their children makes many women feel stronger, thus posing a threat to a controlling man. He might try to reduce the amount of time a mother spends with her children or interfere with the quality of their relationships. He might insist on always being present with the children. Or he might obligate the mother to work extra hours so she cannot be with her children as much as she would like. Or he might insist that he—as a man—should be the one to take the children to certain events rather than the mother.

> Connecting with their children makes many women feel stronger, thus posing a threat to controlling men.

By professing love for the children and becoming their buddies, or conversely by openly rejecting them, or by abusing them, a controlling man builds a wedge between a woman and her children. He might try to persuade the mother that her attachment to her children is unhealthy or unnatural, and interferes with their life as a couple. He might force the woman to choose, constantly, between siding with her child and siding with him, or between spending time with her child and spending time with him. He might deliberately schedule "couple time" for moments when he knows she wants to be with her child. Women sometimes retreat under all this pressure and allow their relationships with their children to deteriorate.

Some men accuse women of being sexually inappropriate with their own sons, whether this son is a child, adolescent, or young adult. This might cause the woman to withdraw from her son. Some controlling men flirt with their partners' daughters. Even if this flirting appears not to be aimed at a goal of eventual sexual abuse, it can still separate a woman from her daughter if it makes one or both of them uncomfortable. A woman's partner should not flirt with her daughter.

An abuser will create rifts between a woman and her child if he plans to sexually abuse that child. The more strained the relationship between the mother and child, the greater the likelihood that he will be able to sexually abuse the child undiscovered. The child feels forced to lie to the mother to cover up the abuse and then grows angry with the mother for failing to protect him or her.

Undermining Her Parenting

A controlling man undermines a woman's parenting by finding ways to become the only authority in the house and encouraging children to disrespect their mother. He may do this subtly by breaking the mother's rules, such as by allowing a child to watch television before doing homework. Sometimes a controlling man will tell children to respect their mother, while at the same time doing whatever he can to reduce her influence in the home. A controlling man undermines a mother by calling her names, criticizing her, or physically abusing her in front of her child. Children come to see the abuser as the source of "real" power and their mother as weak. The children then cease to follow the mother's instructions and seem "out of control," making her feel less and less capable. She may end up hitting and shouting at her children, reinforcing the impression that she is helpless or overly emotional.

> A controlling man tries to become the only authority in the house and encourages children to disrespect their mother.

Often a controlling man imposes his view of parenting and discipline on a woman and her children. This is particularly problematic if he comes in as a stepfather or stepfather figure, and tries to change everything all at once. This is like suddenly forcing a moving vehicle to change directions—it is dangerous.

Jared moved in with Helen and her children just a week after his previous girlfriend had kicked him out of her apartment. Jared responded to Helen's online advertisement for a tenant to rent a room. He almost immediately became Helen's boyfriend, stopped paying rent, and took charge of the household, including the children. He set up elaborate rules for just about everything, including mealtimes, use of the bathroom, and housework. Seeing that Helen was exceptionally close to her 12-year-old daughter, Ariela, Jared was especially strict with her, criticizing and disciplining Ariela almost constantly. Helen would not let Jared hit Ariela, but she watched in angry silence when Jared sent Ariela to her room and made her do sit-ups or write Bible verses as punishment. Helen felt trapped. If she stood up for Ariela, Jared would rage at her. If she allowed Jared to discipline the child, Ariela grew furious at her. Helen felt hopeless about finding a solution, until she met with a professional counselor who helped her persuade Jared to move out, for the good of the children. Shortly after he moved out, Helen decided to end her relationship with him altogether.

Like Jared, many controlling men deliberately disturb a mother's relationship with her children, controlling the children as well as their mother.

Threatening Her Children

An abuser often controls a woman by threatening her children's well-being. The father or father figure may refuse to spend money on a child's medical treatment, clothing, or other expenses, or make the child's mother do specific things if she wishes to support these necessities. He may threaten to take the children and disappear, report the mother to child protective services, or hurt the children.

Children learn to accommodate the behaviors of a controlling man as a survival strategy. To satisfy the adult they perceive as powerful and possibly dangerous, children often laugh at a controlling man's putdowns of their mother and gang up with him against her. Children may be bribed, pushed, or just inspired into degrading or spying on their mother or even hurting her physically. In effect, the children are forced to extend the reach of the controlling man. When children try to take care of and protect their mother, they put themselves at risk.

> To survive, children learn to accommodate the behaviors of a controlling man.

Women often become attached to their partner's children from previous relationships. Controlling men manipulate women through these bonds.

Early in their relationship Fred asked his girlfriend, Terri, to promise his children she would never leave them. The promise did not feel quite right. But because Fred asked her this in front of the children, Terri did not feel that she could refuse. When their relationship as a couple deteriorated and Terri wanted to get as far away from Fred as she could, she felt bound by her promise to the children to try to see them every other week. This forced her to have more contact with Fred than she would have liked. Eventually, she apologized to the children and broke off contact with them, too.

Chapter 7 (pages 125–144) discusses ways to help children cope with their mother's separation from a controlling man.

PART II

Why Coercive Control Happens

Part II explains why coercive control relationships occur. Chapter 3 describes why some men abuse their female partners; society makes it easy for them to do so, and no one stops them. The chapter also discusses individual influences on abusive men, such as their boyhood role models, popular culture, trauma, addictions, and mental illness. Chapter 4 illustrates how women are made vulnerable and the barriers they face as they struggle to free themselves from these relationships. It also describes the countless ways women resist and manage their circumstances, to survive almost impossible conditions.

3

Why Some Men Control Their Partners in This Way

Some men engage in coercive control because they like the feeling of power it gives them. Whether they feel weak or masterful in other areas of their lives, they know they hold power with their partner. Other men are motivated by gender stereotypes where men make the decisions and women do as they are told. Often men convince themselves that they are acting out of pure love. An abuser can get real benefits from coercive control, taking his partner's money and pressuring her to do the housework, cooking, and child care, while he enjoys his "time off" and expects sex on demand. A controlling man intimidates, degrades, manipulates, and monitors his partner so he can reap these benefits.

CHILDREN LEARN THEIR GENDER ROLES

From a young age, most girls learn to be caretakers and most boys expect to be cared for by others. Even today, girls are often expected to cook, clean, nurture their siblings, and generally be pleasing and helpful. In contrast, boys are rarely asked to do household chores other than perhaps clearing their dishes or taking out the trash. Instead of being asked to soothe or adapt to others, boys are often forgiven when they explode emotionally or act rowdy, selfish, or moody. Their behavior is explained and excused. After all, "boys will be boys."

> Young girls learn to be caretakers and most boys expect to be cared for by others.

Women and men carry this early conditioning with them into adulthood. They are primed to enter relationships in an imbalanced way—with women generally doing all they can to keep people calm and pleased and men more focused on getting their own needs met. Women typically do the emotional work of the couple, tending to the relationship and making sure their husbands and children are content. Clearly, this sets up a situation ripe for exploitation by a controlling man.

Most boys are raised to compete with other boys in both friendly and cutthroat ways. They learn to fight, boast, and hurt others to get ahead. In contrast, most girls learn to cooperate, sacrifice for others, and support those around them. These habits show up on the playground, where boys tend to choose rough, vigorous games (or electronic games) with a clear winner and loser. Girls frequently help each other jump rope, play clapping games, or talk about the people in their world. Girls also often join with each other in games of make-believe, enacting scenes of the home life that they've been taught is so key to their future. Children learn to act in these ways by watching the adults around them. Children receive praise for conforming to the expectations of their sex or punishment when they fail to conform.

Although some families and communities teach both boys and girls to be their future husband or wife's best friend and equal partner, traditional values still show up in the media and in religious institutions. People's expectations of their relationships often conform to these ideas more than they realize. The social stereotypes teach a boy that someday he will have a woman whose most important job will be to love and nurture him, while he makes important decisions to guide her and the family. Girls often learn to expect to be taken care of by an all-knowing man. (These ideas are communicated to most children, even those who will someday grow up to live in same-sex relationships.) These expectations set up couples to expect the woman to be loving and the man to be the boss.

Some men carry this early training in competition and domination into their adult lives, acting like bullies at work or on the sports field. Many men find that the easiest person to dominate is their romantic or sexual partner. If a man expects a woman to meet all his needs, then he will not respect her autonomy and will pressure her constantly to build her life around him.

Boys Learn to Control and Abuse

Three individual factors contribute to a man's using coercive control with his partner: First, he has dominating tendencies. Second, he does not respect his partner as a separate human being. And third, he gives himself permission to act in controlling or abusive ways with his partner. Society generally reinforces men for the behaviors and ideas that contribute to using coercive control.

Often controlling men speak to their wives with the same superior, all-knowing, and disrespectful tone that an exasperated parent might use with a child. They learned to use this tone in the families where they grew up.

> **Society generally reinforces men for acting controlling and domineering.**

Some boys whose fathers punish them harshly grow up to punish their own partners and children in similar ways. When he spanks his son, a father is teaching his son that it is okay to hurt others when disappointed or angry. Although it is not his intention, the father is demonstrating that physical force and intimidation help men get their way. The father is also depriving the son of a healthy, positive example: seeing a man resolve his conflicts in a sensible way, without verbal or physical threats. Using corporal punishment, parents teach children that threatening and violent behavior has a place in the family. They are taught that violent actions are justified at times, even with loved ones. As adults, controlling men have no trouble finding the justification to "punish" their wife or girlfriend.

Sometimes a boy who grows up in a home where his father abuses or controls his mother becomes a gentle and kind partner, vowing to avoid the life of his parents. However, often a boy who sees a man control or abuse his mother repeats this behavior with his own girlfriend or wife. He has learned to disrespect and devalue women. His father has modeled for him that it's okay to strike out verbally or physically against the people he loves most and that this is what women deserve.

Popular music and movies frequently glorify men's violence against women and their control over their partners. Reality television programs highlight men who are womanizers in a variety of settings. In the *Real Housewives* series, this misbehavior takes the form of "ladies' men" who can afford multiple women who seem to have little to do with their time other than fret about their looks and spend money. In several television series directed toward African Americans, this takes the form of stories about "players" who have multiple sexual conquests and multiple "baby mamas." Generally, the men in these programs treat women like objects.

Sports figures and other celebrities make headlines for their ability to control women through money, manipulation, and violence. In video games, boys and men often learn to identify with male figures who shoot, sexually assault, torture, restrain, and otherwise torment female characters.

Produced by men for men, most pornography provides lessons in men's total control over women. Real women are hurt in the production of pornography. In addition, the fantasies enacted in pornography combine violence and sex. By consuming pornography, boys and men learn that violence is sexy, sex is violent, and complete control over a woman is the biggest turn-on of all. Women who were sexually victimized by

> Women who were sexually abused by their partners often report that pornography was involved.

their partners often report that pornography was involved in their abuse. Some men tie up or inflict pain on their partners in ways that they first saw enacted in pornographic videos.

By watching these controlling male figures in their families and in the media, boys acquire a distorted vision of what it means to "be a man." Many boys learn to express their desires and distress physically, rather than by voicing their opinions and feelings. Nevertheless, most boys do not grow up to become men who abuse women. Boys see a range of models everywhere for the kind of men they want to be. Two brothers who grow up in the same household might choose different paths. The older brother might model himself on his angry and domineering father, whereas the younger brother might choose to follow in the steps of a kind and gentle uncle or teacher. Abusing a woman is always a choice—men do not simply inherit this tendency from their fathers or acquire it from society.

> Abusing is always a choice—men do not simply inherit this tendency from their fathers or acquire it from society.

THIS MOMENT IN HISTORY

Men dominate women in most major societies today. Men control most of the top positions in finance, politics, entertainment, sports, real estate, science, education, and religion. These positions of authority enable men to retain their privilege over women in public and private life. Men generally earn higher wages and own more property than women. Men are usually larger, stronger, and more physically confident than women, allowing them to intimidate women by their very presence. While most women take great care not to put themselves at risk for assault—by staying home at night and avoiding dark places, for instance—men rarely feel they need to take similar precautions. For all these reasons and more, men and women experience the world differently.

Entire belief systems enshrine men's control over women. Some men use their religious faith as an explanation for their control. Individual men avoid responsibility for their actions by pointing to religious or other doctrines and saying, "You are supposed to obey me." Some women comply with this willingly, some resist, and some reject the doctrine altogether. Most major religions include tenets that are used to oppress women, as well as other tenets that could be used to help women live in freedom.

In addition to traditional influences, various social communities on the Internet advocate men's rule over women. Some treat this kind of relationship as a "lifestyle option." Such websites advance their cause by offering "how-to" information on establishing, maintaining, and enforcing men's control over women in intimate relationships. (Online communities advocating women's dominance over men do exist, but are much less common.) These online communities promote practices ranging from men spanking women to husbands treating their wives as slaves. They support their beliefs with a variety of ideologies, ranging from distorted interpretations of Christianity to antifeminist rhetoric to a kind of "back to the earth" notion that men's "natural" place is to dominate women. Participants in these website discussions request support and advice to help them adopt "the lifestyle" more completely. Many of the females write about their longing for security. They seem to believe that becoming obedient to a man will assure them a lifetime of fidelity and devotion. However, the discussions also reveal trouble in paradise—the relationships described seem to be as marked by betrayals and disappointments as any other relationship. Once they have renounced most goals other than pleasing their partners, the women are unusually dependent and isolated if their relationships fail.

> Most major religions include tenets that oppress women, as well as other tenets that could be used to help women live in freedom.

In societies where the law, religion, and culture all limit women, men do not need to exert coercive control individually to gain obedience. Neighbors and extended family all watch over women and pressure them to conform. Society as a whole restricts women's clothing, movements, and relationships. However, when men move from a place with strong social rules restricting women to a new country with relative freedom, sometimes they panic at their loss of status and power. Those men who cannot make the social adjustment try to push their wives and daughters back into submission, using individual strategies of coercive control, sometimes including violence.

In societies where the law offers women roughly the same liberties as men, those men who wish to control their daughters, girlfriends, and wives try hard to enforce their power directly and frequently. Although physical violence toward women still occurs often, it is increasingly criminalized and frowned on in the United States and other developed countries. Coercive control emerges, then, as the strategy men can still use to control women, without attracting the attention of neighbors or the police.

MEN'S STRUGGLES INFLUENCE THEIR BEHAVIOR

Of course, not every man feels more powerful than every woman. In fact, many abusers feel powerless and frightened. They control others to hide their own feelings of impotence. If an abusive man is unable to control his life or his environment, he might take it out on his wife or girlfriend, to regain a feeling of power. This is especially likely if other people have witnessed his ineffectiveness.

> When men feel disempowered, sometimes they control or abuse the women in their lives to feel more powerful once again.

Jason's father and older brother both worked as electricians and made fun of Jason because he had gone into "clean hands" work, as a salesman. Whenever something mechanical broke, such as the dishwasher or a vacuum, his wife, Sheryl, tried to get it repaired before Jason found out. If Jason knew something was broken, he would try to fix it himself and often failed. He seemed to feel like less of a man because he couldn't fix it. He would grow furious and

*take it out on his wife. Shouting and humiliating Sheryl seemed
to make him feel better again.*

A controlling man who feels emotionally numb might rely
on his partner both for support and for a way to reach his feelings.
When he upsets her, he feels more alive and in control. Paradoxically, while he might degrade her until she cries, he might also
punish her for crying. He forces her to show weakness, but these
signs of weakness make him uncomfortable because they remind
him of how fragile he really is.

Some controlling men have what psychologists call "anxious
attachments." This means they live in fear of being abandoned by
the people who are most important to them. A man who feels this
way needs constant assurance that his wife or girlfriend will love
him and meet his needs, and will not leave him. Such a man will
be unusually alert to any (real or imagined) signs that his partner
is losing interest in him or showing interest in someone else. He
acts possessive and jealous to keep his partner near him. Unfortunately, sometimes these very behaviors drive her away.

Often a controlling man has workmates or drinking buddies
but few true friends. He feels lonely. His worries about the relationship with his wife or girlfriend may lead him to seek constant
reassurance that she will stay with him. If he thinks he sees signs
that she is pulling away, he will punish her because he is deeply
afraid that he could not survive without her. Also, he has trouble
seeing her as a separate person who is free to make the choice to
end the relationship. He acts controlling because he believes this
is the only way to make sure the woman will not abandon him.

Trauma

Some (but certainly not all!) men who have a history of trauma
become suspicious, easily provoked, and controlling. These traits
may have helped the traumatized man stay safe at one time, but
they hinder his ability to relate to his partner. Someone who has

experienced violence in the home, at school, on the streets, or at war may have trouble controlling his feelings and impulses. Everyday events may trigger reactions to the original trauma situation. He may not be aware of this process as it is happening. For example, a man who has been brutalized by his father or in the military might grow violently angry when he feels he is being challenged. (The anger may feel uncontrollable

> **Sometimes a man who has a history of trauma becomes suspicious, easily provoked, and controlling.**

to him, but nevertheless he *can* learn to control it; he is probably regulating his anger already to some degree so that it gets him in as little trouble as possible.)

A trauma history also makes a person more likely to abuse alcohol, street drugs, or prescription medication. This increases his likelihood of behaving badly.

Tyrell returned from his third military deployment nervous and jittery. He had felt okay after the first two deployments, but lifting his buddy's shattered body out of an exploded tank seemed to have pushed Tyrell over an edge. Some days, he didn't want to live. In the war, he lost some of his hearing and suffered a concussion. His back and neck hurt from carrying heavy equipment. But he did not look wounded and he did not want to seek help—he thought complaining was a sign of weakness.

Tyrell took painkillers and smoked cigarettes almost constantly. He worked in the military at a job he considered "boring," putting in his time until he could retire. His family's concerns seemed trivial, and home life seemed superficial and dull, compared to the excitement of war. He felt disoriented and anxious. He knew he was drinking too much.

Tyrell wanted to get everything "in order" again. To accomplish this, he tried to control every aspect of his household. He demanded that his wife and children stick to a rigid schedule and tell him where they were going at all times. Even though he knew it was unlikely, a part of him suspected that his wife had had an affair while he was deployed. He followed her around town to check up on her. He insisted that she wear extremely modest clothes when she was out of the house, but then demanded that she dress sexily for him at home. Tyrell slept fully clothed and with a loaded gun under the bed. Every few days he exploded at his wife. Sometimes he left the house without telling her where he was going. She felt unsafe and as if she could do nothing right.

For some traumatized men, like Tyrell, alcohol and drug abuse help them cope with their trauma symptoms but also contribute to their controlling and explosive ways. Recovering from repeated traumas, like those that occur in war or in childhood abuse, may take years, and many people cannot fully recover. A man with a long or intense trauma history will need to seek professional help focused on the trauma. If he continues to abuse or control his partner, he should not expect her to "stand by his side" while he tries to recover. Some men are able to stop being abusive as they work on their issues.

Past trauma underlies some people's control and abuse. However, these behaviors always involve elements of choice. Abusers need to take responsibility for their actions and stop giving themselves permission to control or hurt their loved ones. In addition, we must remember that most people who control their partners do not act controlling or violent in other situations. They keep themselves in line. Also, while some controlling or violent behaviors may appear impulsive or "out of control," others have been carefully planned. For all these reasons, a history of trauma does not entirely explain controlling or abusive behavior directed only at loved ones. Trauma treatment alone will not automatically reduce a person's violence or his coercive control over his partner.

Someone who has been neglected as a child may have trouble tuning in to another person's needs and may even feel panicky when he grows close to his partner. He has learned that depending on another person is risky. Paradoxically, just when he is feeling closest to his partner, he may push her away or mistreat her.

> A person who was neglected as a child may have trouble tuning in to his partner and may panic when they grow too close to each other.

Alcohol, Drugs, and Mental Illness

Some people who control their partners also abuse alcohol, recreational drugs, or prescription drugs. These substances can make abusers behave more cruelly or violently than usual, but they are not the cause of their controlling behavior. Many people abuse substances without controlling their partners, and many people control their partners without abusing substances. Substance abuse treatment alone will not stop a person from using coercive control. At the same time, an abuser will not be able to do the hard work required to stop controlling his partner until he has overcome his addictions. The bottom line: someone who uses coercive control and also abuses substances needs treatment for both problems.

> A person who uses coercive control and also abuses substances needs treatment for both problems.

A person who is under the influence is less able to control his impulses. He may drive the car extra fast to intimidate his partner, or shout at her louder than usual when he is drunk or high. He may slap her face harder than he intended. However, even at these times, he has not simply lost control—he has given himself permission to act aggressively toward her.

Bill saved his drinking for weekends. He knew his wife, Laurel, was concerned about his drinking and his weight, and he used her concern against her. When Bill was angry, he would pop beer after beer in front of Laurel and chug them down, as if to say, "You try to stop me."

Bill became sloppy and unpredictable when drinking too much. Sometimes he'd grab Laurel in front of the children and insist that she dance with him. Or he would pull her to bed, where he might grow angry with her if he was too drunk to get an erection. At other times, when drunk, he would grow gloomy and critical, telling Laurel that she had ruined his life and he would never amount to anything because of her. Once he took the set of dishes that Laurel had been given by her parents on their wedding day and smashed each plate, frightening Laurel and the children. As usual, Bill left the mess for Laurel to clean up.

Laurel got into the habit of sending the children off to neighbors' houses when Bill began drinking. Over time, Laurel realized that Bill broke only her own possessions when he was drinking— never items that he himself cared about. This led her to suspect that he knew what he was doing, even when drunk. Laurel also noticed that when Bill was with his parents and siblings, he drank a lot but managed to stay in a respectable mood. Laurel began to suspect that Bill drank, in part, to give himself permission to behave cruelly toward her, losing control to gain control. Laurel realized that even if—somehow—Bill was able to stop drinking, he was unlikely to stop his abuse. Laurel started meeting with a counselor at the local women's center to plan a safe way to end the relationship.

A person who is withdrawing, suffering from a hangover, or craving a substance feels terrible. However, in all these situations the abuser is not simply lashing out—he aims his irritability toward a particular person. He targets the woman in his life because he has given himself permission to do so.

Some people who control their partners are suffering from mental illness. For example, clinical depression can make a person quite irritable and short tempered. Someone who is paranoid may express jealousy beyond all reason as well as other fears. A person with obsessive–compulsive disorder may require rigid obedience, enforcing rules that make no sense to others. While suffering from a manic episode, a person might gamble, engage in bizarre sexual behavior, or spend money he does not have. When psychotic, a man might obligate his wife and children to hide from phantoms that he fears, or avoid food that he imagines is poisoned.

However, the control and the mental illness are separate issues. Treating an abuser's mental illness is not likely to stop his controlling attitudes and the acts that follow from these attitudes.

Most men who control women are not mentally ill. Rather, their faulty ideas about themselves and women lead them to take a series of steps that exert control. They may believe these steps are driven by some specific need ("I'd better find out what she's doing") rather than understanding their own more general motivation of exerting control.

WHY SOME MEN WON'T LET GO

Many people wonder why women stay in relationships that include battering or coercive control. The next chapter addresses this question. People seldom ask why *men* stay in these relationships or move from one controlling relationship to another. Often a woman tries to get the controlling man to move out, move on, and leave her alone. But he hangs on like a pit bull, even putting his reputation, career, and family at risk so he

> Why do some men risk their reputation, career and family, to hold on to a woman who wants to leave?

will not have to let go. Some men choose to face jail time or undergo long and expensive divorce trials rather than separate from the women they are trying to control.

Why?

• **Relying on their partners.** Often controlling men are highly dependent on the women in their lives to look after them emotionally as well as physically (keeping house and providing meals and sex). These men typically rely on their partners for feelings of security and wholeness. They are bound to the woman with threads of desperation. They often feel hollow inside and fear a sense of complete emptiness if the tie to the woman is cut. Feeling dependent and vulnerable both frightens and angers them. As much as a man might criticize or degrade his partner, he finds it too painful to ask himself, "Who am I without this woman?" Some men also depend on their women financially and fear that they will be unable to survive financially alone.

• **Fearing failure.** As long as they can maintain their relationship with the woman, they can tell themselves that they are good husbands or boyfriends and good men. Some of these men are successful in their work or other spheres of their lives, while others might be seen as "losers." In either case, they would see separation as an insult to their reputation and self-image. They hang on to women who do not want to be with them because it helps them feel they are winning the battle.

- **Holding distorted ideas of love.** Some men define the habit of being with their partner and the combination of connection and arousal they feel in her presence as love. Like many women, they may also subscribe to romantic ideas about love, including the notion that love lasts forever, losing love is fatal, and love erases the boundaries between two people. These ideas of love can drive men to insist on maintaining their relationship, even when the woman clearly indicates that she wants out.

- **Not knowing how to be in relationships without control.** Some abusers control not only their partners but also their children, friends, and coworkers. They may be willing to obey their bosses. They relate to all others as being above or below them in a hierarchy—and they either give or take orders accordingly. They do not know how to handle a relationship of equals. They will not "let" a woman leave because they insist on being in charge of these sorts of decisions. They will often say something like "The relationship is over when I say it's over."

- **Getting pleasure out of hurting another person.** Women know it when they see it—a man who seems to get a kick out of making her weep, tremble, panic, or bleed. Often, over time, he has to make her hurt worse to get the same buzz of pleasure— whether this is through hitting or sexually assaulting her, restricting her movements, or cutting her down through his words.

Chapter 7 (pages 125–144) discusses stalking and other harassing behavior many abusers employ when their partners try to end the relationship.

Why Some Women Get and Stay Involved

ALL WOMEN ARE VULNERABLE

A woman's education, upbringing, personality, finances, or religion cannot wholly protect her from a controlling relationship, although the right combination may make it easier for her to break free. A woman who crosses paths with a controlling man may find herself caught in his web before she realizes it is a web. Once involved, he will do his best to keep her entangled. Typically, she will try dozens of strategies to regain control of her life, including trying to get away.

> A woman may be caught in the web of an abuser before realizing it is a web.

Certain characteristics in women may initially make them more vulnerable to the advances of a controlling man. Health problems and physical, emotional, and intellectual disabilities make people vulnerable to those who act helpful but have controlling intentions. A woman who has little worldly experience, or one whose family or cultural ideas fit easily with coercive control may be less apt to reject a suitor when his first signs of control appear. Women may be at special risk if they lack money, housing, immigration documents, or other necessary resources. A woman going through a big transition such as leaving her parents' home, graduating school, or getting a divorce may be especially vulnerable. A controlling man will look for and exploit the weaknesses he sees in a particular woman.

Women who previously have been victimized, or who witnessed their mothers being victimized, sometimes have trouble defending themselves against men who would do them harm. They may not recognize when their partner has "crossed the line" and become abusive. These women may have learned to accept as normal the idea that love comes with violence and control. Women who were sexually victimized in their childhood often have trouble asserting their will and defending themselves against future assaults.

Girls who have grown up in poverty and have watched their mothers struggle financially sometimes swear they will find the right partner and keep him happy so he will stick around and help support the household. Financial fears make them unusually determined to make their relationships work, regardless of the personal cost.

Also, a woman cannot think clearly if she is abusing alcohol or other recreational or prescription drugs. Controlling men take advantage of this foggy mind state and use it against their partners. Abusive men often intensify a woman's addictions by encouraging her to take more drugs or experiment with new substances. The less clearly she thinks, the easier it is for him to manipulate her. In the same vein, it may be to his advantage to make sure she is sleep deprived.

However, knowing some of the factors that can make women especially vulnerable should not lead us to think that a woman in a controlling relationship entered that relationship because of a defect or problem in her own psyche. We must be careful to avoid blaming the victim of coercive control or think it is her fault for falling prey to a controlling man. Nor should we think that women who are rich, educated, confident, and trauma-free will necessarily be able to avoid victimization. Some controlling men look for an accomplished woman. She is appealing and has resources he could use.

Ivan was a 45-year-old unemployed businessman. He met 38-year-old Doreen, a highly successful broker, through an online dating service. Ivan sensed that Doreen was eager to get married and have children. Within a year of their meeting, Doreen bought a large apartment for the two of them and gave Ivan money to set up his own business. Ivan spent little time working and was not attentive to Doreen or the son they soon had together. Doreen waited on Ivan and allowed him to boss her around because she felt sorry for him, since he was less successful than she was. Ivan abused Doreen emotionally. No matter how much she gave him and catered to him, it was never enough. He was sarcastic and critical. He showed her no verbal or physical affection after their son was born. When Doreen finally asked Ivan to leave, he threatened to fight for custody of their son. Eventually, Doreen agreed to pay Ivan a large monthly sum so she could keep custody of their child. She supported Ivan economically until their son turned 18.

Women who are smart and successful professionally may be especially determined to make their relationship work. They are used to figuring out problems. They are not accustomed to failure and don't like to back out of difficult situations. They keep trying.

The bottom line: Any woman can fall into a controlling relationship. Women with fewer resources have a harder time breaking free.

TRAPPED BY ROMANCE, LOVE, AND CONFUSED FEELINGS

Most relationships that become controlling and destructive do not appear that way at the beginning. At first the abuser may seem like the partner the woman has been seeking—devoted, loving, supportive, and wanting to spend every minute together.

Women are often overcome with feelings of love, romance, and optimism as they enter these intense and intoxicating relationships. They may be swept into an altered state where reality seems suspended. Over time, a controlling man produces a range of confused feelings in his victim, including fear, love, shame, and dependence. All these feelings make it difficult for her to leave, even as the relationship deteriorates. She keeps trying to please her man, hoping she can once again bask in his earlier pure, loving gaze. Controlling men harness these romantic impulses and strong feelings, using them to make women submit and stay.

Most controlling men sprinkle in moments of romance, love, and connection together with their cruelty and control. During these brighter times of kindness and support, the woman feels cared for and loved. His kindness is like a glass of water for a thirsty traveler. She wants it so much! It feels so good! His strategy of occasionally rewarding her keeps her compliant, and she sticks around, hoping for more. It is the same process that makes people gamble or check obsessively for messages on their cell phones, social networking pages, and e-mail accounts—occasionally they are rewarded with something they really like. Even in controlling and abusive relationships, a woman sees bright spots and hopes things will improve.

In recent decades people have thought of men's physical violence against their partners as being cyclical, with an episode of violence followed by a honeymoon period in which the abuser tries to woo her back. Then there is a phase when the abuser acts as if nothing has happened or makes light of the incident. This in turn is followed by a period of building tension in which the woman tries to avoid provoking her partner. This process is often called "the cycle of violence." Drawings of this cycle appear on the websites of most organizations that work with partner violence.

However, these periods of kindness appear different when seen through the lens of coercive control. The recurring honeymoon or acts of kindness are part of the same controlling strategy as the episodes of anger or physical violence—just another tactic.

The woman may welcome the roses, kisses, and compliments, believing these are signs that her partner is changing. However, the kinder periods are ploys to make her stay. The abuser chooses to act kindly when he believes that expressing love is the best strategy for retaining control. Sure, he may genuinely want to connect with her. He may love her. But more than anything, these periods of kindness work to keep the woman hopeful and coming back for more.

> Occasional acts of kindness are a strategy to retain control and make a partner stay in the relationship.

Roberta would deny that Anton, her husband of 20 years, was violent. Sometimes he grabbed her arms a little too hard. And every few months he insisted that they have what he called "wild sex," even though he knew it hurt her. Occasionally he'd stomp his foot or punch a wall when he was angry. Sometimes he'd "get up in her face" and speak loudly and slowly, pointing his finger and making her feel like a little girl being scolded by her cruel father. She'd usually cry and feel ashamed. But they had good times, too, with their children and their circle of family and friends. After he had been especially nasty to her, Anton would shower Roberta with flowers and compliments. He'd take her out to her favorite restaurant. He would pull her onto the couch to look at their wedding album and tell Roberta she was just as pretty today as the day they had met, when he knew they'd be together for the rest of their lives. Roberta felt bound to Anton by her love for him and her commitment, as well as by traces of fear.

For women like Roberta, submitting to a man's hostile and violent behaviors can grow to seem routine. She struggles to preserve her self-esteem and keep herself safe by doing whatever her partner wants. The ways she accommodates him may keep the peace in the short term. In the long term, they make her more isolated and less free.

When a woman lives with a man's physical and verbal violence, she sometimes develops a traumatic bond with him, similar to the bond that hostages can develop with their captors. He gives her enough kindness and pleasure to keep her attached. After shouting, he may comfort her, which she comes to see as an enormous gift. She adopts his values, ignores her own needs, and feels safe as she grows closer and closer to the very source of danger.

Seen from afar, it might seem obvious that a woman should break free from a partner who is abusive or overly controlling. We must remember that the situation looks different when a woman is in the middle of it. She focuses on the details. On any given day she is apt to note what went well and what went poorly in the relationship without noting her partner's overall controlling intention. Some of his behaviors look like ways he is supporting her (to lose weight or to make better use of her time, for instance); some look like signs of the intensity of his love (expressions of jealousy, wanting to be with her at all times); and some may look like simple quirks or even responses to her mistakes. Although hindsight is often 20/20, people who are in the throes of a relationship can rarely assess it accurately.

> **Traumatic bonds sometimes develop between a victim and an abuser, similar to the bond between a hostage and a captor.**

Over time in a relationship of coercive control, the victim experiences confused feelings, distorted thoughts, and a numbness or paralysis that makes leaving more difficult. She often feels drained and despairing.

Like many women in similar situations, Genie reported feeling hopeless. "Staying is killing me," she said, "but getting out would also kill me for sure."

Controlling men manipulate their partners' feelings so their wives and girlfriends end up isolating and restricting themselves. As the women become increasingly solitary and lose self-esteem, they may have trouble imagining themselves living apart from their partner. The woman may feel a general sense of dread, and lose the confidence that could help her strike out on her own. She may come to believe that she cannot live without her man.

Many people are confused about the relationship between love, control, and jealousy. They believe that when you love a person deeply, jealousy follows; and jealousy leads naturally and inevitably to attempts to control the other person. So if the controlling person says, "I won't let you go downtown alone because I love you so much and it makes me jealous to think of all those men looking at you," or "Give me your e-mail passwords so I can see that you are not writing other men," his word rules. And he may truly be suffering, tormented by the notion that his partner's attentions are wandering. If the woman objects to these constraints as overly controlling, she is told they are signs of love. One of the hallmarks of coercive control is that the controlling person gets to define reality. If he says it's "love," then it's "love," even if it feels like control.

> The controlling person defines reality. If he says it's "love," then it's "love," even if it feels like control.

TRAPPED BY GENDER EXPECTATIONS

Girls today face mixed messages about how they should live their lives. Their schools and even some family members stress the importance of a career and financial independence. At the same time, popular movies, songs, books, and magazines show romantic love as the key to lasting happiness.

Romantic comedies routinely show two mismatched people who conquer great obstacles to find lasting love. She is always a beauty, and he is often beastlike in some way, before she transforms him into the man of her dreams. In these movies the man's behavior often troubles and confuses his future mate until the misunderstanding melts away and they live happily ever after. The courtship is bumpy, but the dream of perfect love is their prize.

A woman who commits strongly to the idea of "true love until the end" may find it difficult to assert herself when problems arise in a relationship with a controlling man. An abuser takes advantage of this romantic commitment, framing conflict as her fault and as a threat to the relationship. His words and actions communicate something like this: "If you cared about us as a couple, you wouldn't make problems." Women keep silent to avoid making waves.

> A controlling person communicates: "If you cared about us as a couple, you wouldn't make problems." Women keep silent to avoid making waves.

Hannah was 20 and in her third year of college when she met Drake, 28. He was manager at the café where she worked part-time. Drake asked Hannah to go dancing with him. They had great chemistry. Drake told Hannah he was old-fashioned and wanted to save sex for marriage. He kissed her briefly but passionately when he took her back to her dorm after their date.

Soon they spent every weekend evening together. Four months later Drake proposed to Hannah dramatically on one knee, with flowers in hand. Hannah accepted and they held a small wedding a month later. They decided they would wait to have children until Hannah had completed her college degree.

After the wedding Drake changed. He assigned her shifts only when he was at the café so they could be together most of the time. One evening he grew angry when Hannah came home later than usual after class, although she had called and said she would be going out with her sister. He said he did not want her staying out late at night, and she should drink alcohol only with him. One day Hannah realized that some of her clothes were missing. When she asked Drake, he told her that he had thrown them out. She would not need to "dress like a hussy" now that she was married.

Drake offered to give Hannah the passwords to his phone and social media accounts and demanded hers. When Hannah objected, Drake called her "paranoid" and questioned her commitment to their marriage.

Even today a woman's primary life project, according to many cultures, is to live in partnership with a man, raise children, and create a happy home. Many women are so committed to this plan that they put up with almost constant oppression, anguish, and discomfort so they will not have to feel like failures. Knowing about a woman's early socialization helps us understand why she would tolerate coercive control; she is working hard to make the relationship succeed and to keep her partner happy.

Some men twist to their own advantage this idea about what it means to be a woman. While coercive control takes different shapes in different cultures, a man's domination of his partner rarely looks entirely out of place in any cultural context. Coercive control is an extreme version of cultural norms that many women face across the globe—norms that place a man's comfort, achievement, and sexual satisfaction far ahead of a woman's.

TRAPPED BY CARETAKING

Controlling men often consider themselves victims and try to evoke women's pity and compassion. Some controlling men have indeed suffered in the past— horrible things happen to many people. It is notable, however, how rarely controlling men take responsibility for their actions and failures, usually blaming someone else.

> Controlling people often consider themselves victims, evoking their partner's pity and compassion.

When a woman becomes involved with a controlling man, she often accepts the stories he tells her as true. She tries to make up for his previous disappointments and becomes his caretaker. She invests in his well-being. He makes her feel needed. She may believe she can help him overcome his problems and realize his potential, despite those who are against him. Typically, she sympathizes with him and cannot bear to see him suffer. Slowly or suddenly, she sacrifices her own well-being to boost his.

When Shana met Jorge, he seemed overwhelmed with caring for his two young children, who he said had been abandoned by their drug-addicted mother. Shana began babysitting Jorge's children in the evening twice a week when he worked overtime. Soon Shana also stayed with the children when Jorge went out at night with friends because he "needed to blow off steam." Jorge would come home tipsy from these evenings with his buddies and expect Shana to have sex with him. Although Shana loved Jorge and the children, she began to feel like a babysitter, cook, and sex worker with Jorge, who kept asking her for a "little more support" because he was going through a difficult time. The children's mother, Cindy, called one day when Jorge wasn't home. Cindy told Shana that she adored her children and desperately wanted to be with them, but had been outmaneuvered by Jorge and his lawyer. Shana was unsettled by the conversation, wondering how much of what Jorge had told her were lies.

Like Shana, when a woman is in love and believes in her man, she often makes his happiness and success her personal project. She believes she can help him change the course of his life. She believes she sees the goodness in him that others miss because he reveals certain sides of himself to her alone. She believes he is a good person who just needs some support. Seeing him as wounded, she doesn't want to get him in trouble so she hesitates to report him to the police or tell anyone about the abuse and control.

Certainly many women help men make important changes in their lives. But if a person does not take responsibility for his actions and simply blames them on others, his situation is unlikely to change. A woman's efforts to help a man improve his life should not require sacrificing her own well-being.

Women also often end up caring for their partner's parents and children from prior relationships. To end a controlling relationship a woman may need to break ties with children and in-laws whom she has grown to love. Raised to be caretakers, many women find it tough to break these bonds.

TRAPPED BY CIRCUMSTANCES

A victim's thoughts explain just a small portion of the process of getting trapped in a relationship of coercive control. A woman who is being coercively controlled is trapped by her circumstances—not by her character. The decision to continue the relationship is not entirely in her hands. Some women depend on their partners financially and in other ways and doubt that they will be able to start over or survive on their own. As a society, we do not offer the supports a woman needs to live on her own, especially if she has children. (These missing supports include affordable housing and healthcare, paid maternity and family leave, subsidized child care, guarantees of a living wage, equal pay for equal work, and so on. All these supports help women achieve financial independence.) Even when courts rule in a victim's favor and it looks as if "everything is working for her," abusers are often skilled at manipulating the system. An abuser might delay child support so long that his victim becomes homeless or desperate enough to go back to him.

> Victims of coercive control are trapped by their circumstances—not by their character.

Women who contemplate ending their relationships face great social pressures and may fear being the target of gossip. They may have been led to believe that their children need a father at all costs. Religious leaders who lack knowledge of coercive control may push women to stay in their oppressive marriages, failing to consider the toll it is taking on the women.

Some women in controlling relationships fear being pushed away by their families, communities, or children if they seek separation or divorce. Cultural and religious ideas often make it difficult for women to end their marriages or defy their partners. Some women have been threatened with deportation, homelessness, or losing custody of children if they end the relationship. Women who are military dependents might face losing their housing, health insurance, children's school, and their access to a pension if they end their marriage.

Annie and Gabriel met in the Army, where they were both active duty officers. They married and continued with their military service. When they decided to have children, Annie considered these challenges: her husband had a flight school commitment and could not get out of the army for eight more years; military members are often deployed away from home for many months at a time; and even when they're not deployed, the military does not guarantee that military spouses will be assigned to the same duty location.

For the sake of her family, Annie left the Army and stayed home with their children. Her status instantly changed from military officer to military "dependent," which she discovered left her disempowered in relation to her husband.

Annie suffered for years from Gabriel's verbal outbursts, insults, and control. Even as she became aware of her husband's multiple extramarital affairs, Annie felt compelled to stay with him. In the tight confines of the military base where they lived, and because her husband was an officer, Annie felt obligated to maintain the illusion of a happy family. She talked to no one about her problems and tried to keep peace at home. She wanted to ensure that her husband's career would not be affected by his behavior. If Gabriel left the military or was kicked out before 20 years of service, the entire family would lose their income, pension, and health care benefits.

When her children grew to be 10 and 12 years old, Annie realized that while she could try to hide her husband's behavior from the outside world, she could no longer hide it from their children. Their son's grades were slipping and he, too, began having angry outbursts. Their daughter was growing withdrawn and fearful.

Annie required a great deal of courage to extricate herself and her children from Gabriel and their military life. Fortunately, although she had no current work experience, Annie's premilitary training enabled her to find a job with her own health insurance *and retirement plan. Other military dependents may have fewer options.*

TRAPPED BY VIOLENCE AND THREATS

In additional to real financial stress, women often fear that their partners will violently assault or even murder them if they separate. Indeed, women are more likely to be killed by their partners during the process of ending a relationship than at any other time.[3] Therefore, a woman who believes it is safer to stay with her abuser than leave him may be assessing her situation accurately. She will need to work out a detailed safety plan so she can exit the relationship safely. A history of coercive control (threats, forcible rape, constant jealousy) is an even better predictor of violence at the point of separation than a history of previous violence (see "Assessing Lethality," pages 137–138). Controlling men cannot bear to have a relationship taken away from them against their will—some act out violently in response.

A woman may try to escape from the relationship multiple times, but her partner will not let her go. He tracks her down, threatens her, beats her, rapes her, and bankrupts her. He might persuade a court to award him custody of the children, even if he has never before been involved in their day-to-day lives. Through his charm and connections, he is often able to manipulate the legal system and the police. Friends, family, and employers may support him and condemn her, not realizing they are being manipulated in a power play (see "Ending the Relationship," pages 156–179).

MANAGING THE UNMANAGEABLE

Women in coercive relationships do not welcome or passively tolerate this control and abuse. Once they feel trapped in such a relationship, most women do everything in their power to improve it and end the problems. Typically, they try to leave numerous times. Even if they stay in the relationship, they are not consenting to its harmful features.

A victim of coercive control usually does what she can to protect herself and her children, making the best of the situation. Typically, she submits to her partner's demands, even as these demands become more exacting, burdensome, and hard to follow. She keeps trying to please him, thinking that if she can only do what he wants a little better, he will be satisfied and become more loving. She may also try to reason with her partner, wanting him to see that he is wrong or is asking too much. She tries to remain hopeful, managing her disappointment by lowering her own expectations. Over time, he may not need to control her in obvious ways—she has learned to conform to his restrictions even without constant pressure.

> A victim of coercive control struggles to keep the peace and protect her family by submitting to the abuser's demands.

Grace resolved, again and again, to continue improving herself so she could please her critical and demanding husband, Arthur. She took cooking lessons and kept her children well behaved. Grace dieted and wore the clothes she knew Arthur preferred. Grace tried to display a pleasing attitude at all times and create an upbeat feeling in her home. She knew that showing a positive disposition would please Arthur's extended family and their church, as well as Arthur himself.

Despite years of trying, Grace's efforts failed. Arthur would sometimes praise her. But he continued to criticize her frequently, demand more from her, and punish her when he felt she had not been trying hard enough. Early in their life as a couple, Arthur told Grace not to leave the house without his permission. Over time, she developed strong fears about going out into the world and stayed home except when he was with her. Arthur no longer needed to restrict Grace—he even mocked her for her fears in front of their children. Grace's anxiety kept her home where he wanted her.

A controlling man will often lead his wife or girlfriend to believe *she* is doing things wrong—things that are in her control—and therefore she is responsible for their problems and deserves the criticism or punishment that he heaps on her. She will often second-guess herself, trying to figure out ways to avoid triggering his disapproval and trying to make amends. He may respond to her neutral or even positive comments as if they were criticisms. A woman in a coercive relationship tends to seek the gentlest way to express herself, to avoid stirring her partner's anger. She may repeatedly consider how to approach her partner without provoking him, and then she is disappointed when these strategies fail. Somehow he still ends up angry with her or disappointed in her. A victim's efforts to please her abuser may look like passive compliance. But in truth she is trying hard to manage or end the violence and control.

> An abuser leads his victim to believe that she is doing things wrong and is responsible for their problems.

RESISTING EVERY DAY: CONTROL IN THE CONTEXT OF BEING CONTROLLED

Most women bravely manage their situations despite great pressures, and many try to leave or get the abuser to leave, again and again.

Most women who are being victimized by a controlling man do not accept their situation passively. For a time, they may be so engulfed in the abuser's reality that they don't notice how their own will is being limited. As months and years go by, however, they grow uncomfortable and seek outlets where they can feel like themselves. If isolated, they typically reach out for ways to make friends. As in a game of cat and mouse, the abuser seeks to eliminate such contacts.

> Most victims bravely manage their situations, and many try to leave or get the abuser to leave, again and again.

Many people who are victimized will go to great lengths to maintain or regain their autonomy through setting up "safety zones." These may be physical places where they feel they can be themselves, or relationships where they feel valued, or hobbies where they can express themselves, or even subtle ways of defying the abuser's wishes.

Safety zones are places or relationships in which a victimized person feels valued and free.

For example, isolated women sometimes use disposable phones or make calls at work, so their abuser cannot track all their contacts. They store money away and hide "unauthorized" purchases. They set up post office boxes, write in journals, secretly use birth control, and meet friends in out-of-the-way places.

Betty completed her college degree online, without her husband's knowledge, so she would have a career to rely on when she escaped.

Lin incorporated her anger and struggle into her artwork, which looked to her husband like a harmless hobby.

Anastasia worked out for a couple of hours each day; shaping her body made her feel healthy and powerful. Her husband controlled her life in many ways, but she was staking a claim to the territory within her skin.

Young Hee slipped words and phrases in Korean into her conversations and e-mails. She suspected her boyfriend was monitoring her communications, and she knew this would frustrate him.

Cynthia hummed gospel hymns from her childhood as she cooked and did housework. They reminded her of happier times, and they helped her maintain her faith that someday she would be free.

Tania placed her children on a waiting list for subsidized child care. As soon as they were accepted, she left her husband.

Georgia met secretly from time to time for coffee with a male friend. They flirted. Sometimes she felt ashamed, but at other times she thought this contact with an appreciative man was the only way she could keep feeling human.

While these examples are all quite different, they show how people turn toward freedom even under oppressive conditions, just as a sunflower always turns toward the sun.

The desire to be able to think and act independently seems to be part of the human condition. Certainly, cultures vary in how much they value independence versus interdependence. In many cultures women are traditionally expected to put their husband's, father's, and brother's interests ahead of their own. However, even in conditions that approach slavery, every human being—male and female—strives to maintain a sense of self. Where they are being controlled by others, whether these others are husbands, bosses, warlords, or pimps, women will sing songs in their minds or recall memories and dreams that allow them to maintain a sense of "This is who I am. This is ME."

People who are victimized by coercive control do not allow themselves to be erased.

PART III

Coercive Control
in Specific Populations

This entire book is designed for people of all genders, sexual orientations, ages, and cultures affected by coercive control. However, people's identities and backgrounds do influence how coercive control shows up in their lives. The following two chapters discuss the special issues affecting LGBT people, men who are victimized by women, and teenage victims of coercive control.

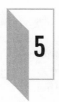

Different Gender Arrangements and Coercive Control

In most coercive control relationships, men dominate women. This is because most couples are heterosexual and society supports men dominating women. However, relationships of coercive control exist outside this more typical arrangement. This entire book is relevant to people of all genders in all kinds of relationships, despite the use the pronouns he/she in most examples. This chapter examines coercive control in the relationships of lesbian, gay, bisexual, and transgender people, and in heterosexual couples where women control their male partner.

LGBT PEOPLE FACING COERCIVE CONTROL

In coercive control relationships, one person tries to control the other's thoughts, feelings, and behaviors. The controller intimidates and punishes to get his or her way. The traditional gender setup of heterosexual relationships facilitates men's coercive control of women. Many people assume that same-sex couples are "naturally" more equal because they lack the male/female stereotypes and history of straight couples. However, some people in same-sex relationships also exert coercive control over their partners. People who are transgender—that is, individuals who do not fall neatly into the traditional categories of male and female—are vulnerable in many of the same ways as gay men and lesbians. As members of a stigmatized group, their partners may have extra power over them.

LGBT people who are victims of coercive control may find themselves especially alone. Some have been disowned by their families for being LGBT and some have kept their sexual orientation or gender identity secret, making it difficult to turn to family members for support. If they live in an area with a relatively small LGBT community, it may be hard to start a new life apart from their abusive ex-partner. They run into the former partner or the former partner's close friends regularly.

> **LGBT victims of coercive control may find themselves especially alone.**

When LGBT victims of coercive control reach out for help within their communities, they may discover that some friends prefer to ignore or deny the problems, acting as if only heterosexual and nontransgender people use violence and control in relationships.

Sarita lived with her partner of a decade, Brenda. In a four-year period, Sarita gave birth to two children, whom she and Brenda planned to raise together. Sarita had previously worked as a teacher, but Brenda persuaded her to stay home with their young children. Rather quickly after the birth of their second child, Brenda started going out to bars after work and arriving home drunk. Brenda began spending time with a former girlfriend, although she denied they were romantically or sexually involved. Whenever Sarita tried to raise her concerns, Brenda told her to stop nagging. Once, Brenda told her, "I've got to get out of here or I'm going to slap you," and did not return until dinnertime the following night, when she acted as if nothing had happened. Although some of Sarita's lesbian friends were supportive, others laughed and told her that she shouldn't be surprised—that since Brenda was "more macho than most men," such behavior should be expected.

LGBT victims of coercive control and abuse are sometimes silenced by other LGBT people. Speaking out about control and violence might be seen as furthering stereotypes and attracting negative attention to a community that is already stigmatized.

Some lesbians have difficulty recognizing control and abuse in their relationships. Lesbian relationships are thought to be "naturally" egalitarian. When a woman feels victimized by another woman, she may doubt her perceptions. She may wonder how she can be victimized with no man present to exert domination. Lesbians may also have special difficulty recognizing sexual coercion and violence in their relationships, since sexual misconduct is thought to be perpetrated only by men.

Societal prejudices against LGBT people make those who are victims of coercive control vulnerable in additional ways. If the controlled person has not publicly disclosed his or her sexual orientation or gender identity, the abuser can threaten to "out" the victim if he or she does not comply with the abuser's demands— putting jobs and friendships at risk. In places where rights are not clearly established for LGBT parents, the abuser may threaten to deny the partner contact with children they have raised jointly. Similarly, in situations where property rights are not accorded fairly to LGBT partners, a controlling person can use economic threats to manipulate his or her partner. If one partner is undocumented, the controlling partner can threaten to tell authorities about his or her immigration status.

Often, LGBT people have had unpleasant encounters with those who should be helping and protecting them: the police, courts, educators, and mental health and medical professionals. This history of discrimination may make them especially hesitant to turn to authorities for help. In addition, professional services are often lacking for LGBT victims of relationship violence. Many domestic violence shelters fail to meet the needs of people hurt in same-sex relationships; some will admit lesbians who are victims but have no facilities for victimized men or transgender people.

Some psychotherapists, clergy, and family members are ignorant about these issues and try to push LGBT people to question their own sexual orientation or gender identity when a relationship fails. However, the problem is not in the person's orientation or identity; it's in the specific controlling relationship.

As with all couples, a large difference in physical size, strength or ability, age, social status, or wealth might make an LGBT person especially vulnerable to coercive control. A certain lack of balance may be part of the "deal" a couple strikes in the beginning of their relationship, where one partner is richer or in some other way more powerful than the other. The less powerful partner may feel fortunate—at least at first—to be able to benefit from the other's wealth or status. Over time, the power differential shows up as abusive control.

Kevin was a 19-year-old undergraduate when he met Steve, 45, his art history professor. They became lovers. Steve soon invited Kevin to move into his architect-designed home. Kevin was happy to get out of the dorms and live rent free. Over the next two years, Kevin discovered that living with Steve came at a price. Steve expected Kevin to do most of the cooking and all the cleaning. Steve expected that Kevin would do whatever Steve wanted sexually every day. Steve would not allow Kevin to bring his friends to the house. When Steve's friends visited, Kevin was expected to cook for them and serve them. Kevin felt as if Steve's friends were laughing at him, seeing him as a sort of mistress. Steve was unwilling to discuss or change their arrangement. In fact, he became more rigid over time about his expectations for Kevin and his restrictions on Kevin's freedom. Eventually, Steve told Kevin to move out, without an explanation, leaving Kevin to feel that he had been Steve's plaything for a couple of years and nothing more.

Sometimes LGBT couples fall into butch–femme roles, where one partner holds a job and takes out the trash while the other stays home, cooks and cleans house, and is responsible for sexually satisfying the wage earner. There is nothing inherently wrong with this kind of relationship, as long as both people feel free and satisfied. The problems come when one partner exploits, traps, threatens, abuses, or controls the other.

Gay men may have trouble recognizing sexual coercion, exploitation, and abuse in their relationships. Being willing to experiment sexually is expected in some communities of gay men. An abuser can push past a partner's boundaries, cloaking his controlling practices as fun exploration that the victim is just "too uptight" to enjoy.

The difficulties discussed here for lesbian, gay, and bisexual populations in general may be more intense for transgender people. Getting "outed" to friends, family, and employers presents great risk to many transgender people who have hidden their status— giving abusers an additional way to control them. In some communities, transgender people risk losing custody of their children or of children they have helped raise with their partner, simply because they are transgender. Transgender people may also face difficulties finding a romantic partner who accepts them. So when a partner says, "no one else will ever love you," the transgender victim may be especially likely to believe this is true and feel trapped.

LGBT victims of coercive control struggle to seek their freedom, like all people in similar situations. The suggestions in Part IV will be helpful to all who are victims of coercive control, regardless of their sexual orientation or gender identity.

WOMEN USING COERCIVE CONTROL WITH THEIR MALE PARTNERS

In most situations of coercive control and intimate partner violence, it's men who control and abuse women.* Occasionally, though, women do systematically dominate their male partners,

---

*Women's use of force in heterosexual relationships rarely includes intimidation, isolation, or threat—hallmarks of coercive control. Men whose female partners have used force with them rarely report living in fear, and the men rarely need to seek medical attention. Most often, women in heterosexual relationships use physical force when involved in a mutual couple fight or in violent resistance, a response to control and usually battering (see page 33). Rarely, a woman who has suffered violence in a previous relationship brings her unresolved issues with her to the new relationship and may become violent.

with or without physical violence. For coercive control to work without the support of the usual gender roles of men over women, the dominating woman typically has some substantial advantage such as greater social status, wealth, or physical mobility.[4] Sometimes men who feel they have been "lifted up" from poverty by their wives will submit to their wives' control. Sometimes the man happens to be unusually gentle and kind, and his partner uses this against him. Or a man submits because he has a physical or psychological disability that makes him vulnerable.

Jerome was in a wheelchair because of a car accident. He was unable to move his legs and had only minimal control over his arms and fingers. At a concert he met and fell in love with Aida, who seemed to adore him passionately. But she also "had a temper." She moved into his apartment within a week after their first meeting. Quickly, she took over the household. Jerome turned over his disability checks to her. Soon he felt like a prisoner. She had canceled the aides who had been coming to help him. This left him isolated. If he did not do what she asked, including signing checks, she would refuse to bathe him and delay giving him meals or water to drink. She criticized and humiliated Jerome, telling him he was worthless and less than a man, because he "couldn't even stand up." Jerome's disability made him vulnerable to physical, psychological, and economic control by a woman.

Some men may tolerate coercive control in their intimate relationships because they feel they have no choice or they have too much to lose if they break away, such as losing access to their children. They may not recognize that they are in an abusive relationship because their relationship does not fit within the typical gender pattern. They may also feel too embarrassed and humiliated to seek help—ashamed of being subject to a woman's control.

Below is an example of a couple with a bossy and abusive woman. Despite the power imbalance, we can see that it does not meet the full criteria for coercive control.

José, from a professional family in Ecuador, met Rita in one of his university classes. A year later, they were engaged. They were both delighted to be moving out of their parents' homes and into their own apartment. They agreed they would wait to have children until they were established professionally.

Once they had married and moved in, Rita insisted that they pool their money. She paid for their household expenses out of their joint account and gave José a small amount of spending money each Monday. She began to track his whereabouts and sometimes waited for him after work to see whom he was speaking with as he left the building.

When in public, Rita sometimes hissed insults or commands between her teeth at José, all the while smiling and keeping up appearances. When alone, she sometimes banged on José with her fists. José found this to be annoying and upsetting, but he did not feel physically threatened. Once Rita started banging on his arms while he was driving and sent his eyeglasses flying. José parked the car. He told her, "Never hit me again," and she didn't.

José was too embarrassed by the hostile situation to tell anyone. The sweet woman he had married had apparently vanished. He kept hoping things would improve. Two years later, after a disastrous vacation, Rita told him she was pregnant. José remained in the marriage for more than a decade, until their two daughters were in middle school.

In this example, we see a man who is in some ways controlled and abused by his wife. But José was not afraid of Rita. He was able to establish limits. She did not punish him other than to shout or refuse to have sex. Although Rita controlled José's spending money, he was not isolated. He continued to work and retained his self-esteem through his job and through friendships he gained by playing soccer.

Because they do not have the societal supports of sexism, women are rarely able to exert full coercive control over their male partners.

6

Teenage Victims
of Coercive Control

This chapter focuses on special issues affecting teenagers in coercive control relationships. Some teens are caught in these relationships when they are quite young, maybe even 12 or 13. Teens can be victimized by partners who are slightly younger, the same age, slightly older, or substantially older. A large age difference increases the likelihood that the younger person will have less power in the relationship.

Because younger teens usually live with their parents or another caretaker, the problem of control may be more limited than in adult relationships—affecting certain but not all aspects of the victim's life. Also, teenage relationships often do not last long, so control and isolation do not have time to deepen. As a result, although many teen relationships do have controlling features, they rarely add up to a full picture of coercive control. Nevertheless, the victim can suffer serious harm.

Some teens are absolutely victims of coercive control. These relationships can make the teens miserable for months or years of their young lives and have highly destructive long-term effects. Through these early pairings, young people learn what it means to be in a relationship and may repeat the same patterns throughout their lives. Also, these early controlling relationships sometimes result in long-lasting outcomes such as low self-esteem, eating disorders, sexually transmitted infections, bodily injury, pregnancy, dropping out of school, early marriage, addictions, and legal and mental health problems.

TEENAGERS' VULNERABILITIES

Typically, teenagers have little experience in romantic or sexual relationships, making it difficult for them to differentiate between a healthy relationship and a problematic one. If something doesn't feel right, they may not trust their feelings. A teenage girl, in particular, will often go along with her boyfriend's demands, trying to minimize conflict. If she tries to assert herself, she faces being labeled "pushy" or worse.

Teens have limited control over their lives. Usually, a parent or other caretaker makes important decisions for teens regarding where they live, where they go to school or work, the medical care they receive, and so on. Teens often hesitate to tell adults about violence and control in their relationships because they don't want the adults to take over. Teens may not know a safe source of help or information, especially if they are afraid of their parents. For these reasons and others, teenagers may have special difficulty getting out of relationships of coercive control.

Frequently, teenage girls are afraid of getting their abusive and controlling boyfriends "in trouble" for violence, for drug use or other illegal behavior, or for statutory rape. Often, like some adult women, they want the relationships to continue, even though they want the violence and the coercive control to stop.

> Teenage victims of coercive control often fear getting their boyfriends in trouble for violence, drug use, or statutory rape.

Teenagers differ widely from each other. Their religious, ethnic, and cultural backgrounds will partially shape their ideas about how they should act in a couple. While a teen's age certainly does not indicate how mature that person might be, a 13-year-old is clearly quite different from a 19-year-old. A teen who attends school lives a far different life from one who has dropped out. Those who hold jobs have different vulnerabilities from those who don't need to work or are unemployed, or those who engage in illegal activities, such as selling drugs.

A teenager who has access to a stable home and parental support may find it easier to avoid or escape from a controlling relationship. On the other hand, escape is especially difficult for a teen who has fled into the arms of an abuser to find relief from homelessness or an unhappy family life. Sadly, through abuse at the hands of a relative or neighbor, some teens have learned to submit to another person's will, and to keep quiet about it. Physical, sexual, or emotional abuse at home often conditions teenagers to submit to their abusive intimate partners outside the home.

Teenagers tend to be romantic, and they have trouble projecting realistically into the future. A controlling teen can cultivate in his partner the idea that the two of them are alone against the world.

If adults disapprove of a young woman's partner because he is older or because he comes from a different ethnic or racial group, social class, or religion, she may feel especially determined to keep the relationship going, despite the control, to prove to the doubters that she was correct in her assessment of him.

Seventeen-year-old Joni met 23-year-old Nessim while both worked at a fast food restaurant one summer. Both sets of parents were angry about the relationship because Joni was a Christian and Nessim was a Muslim. Joni's parents also objected because Nessim was so much older and had not attended college. Joni dropped out of school at the end of the summer, moved in to Nessim's rented room, and continued at the restaurant. She was determined to prove her parents wrong about the relationship. However, shortly after moving in, Joni began to regret her decision. Nessim was obliging her to dress modestly and to avoid situations other than work where she would meet unrelated men, saying it was part of his religion. However, Joni noticed that Nessim drank alcohol and seemed to have no problem interacting with unrelated women. Joni felt she could not end the relationship or speak with her parents about what had happened because they would blame her for her decisions.

People who worry that a young person is entering a destructive relationship should do everything they can to maintain contact and keep communication open.

> Maintain contact and keep communication open with young people who are in a destructive relationship.

ISOLATION, STALKING, AND POSSESSIVENESS

Most teens lack direct experience of peer love relationships. Their parents loved them and exerted control over them, so they may expect that love comes with control. Of course, this is even more common among teens who have seen their mothers controlled by their fathers or father figures or who were abused by a parent themselves as children.

A controlling teenage boy may try to separate his girlfriend from her other friends, either by monopolizing her time or by badmouthing her friends and insisting that she "drop" them. Given how unstable teen friendships can be, once a young woman loses her friends, she may feel that she has lost social standing and will be without friends forever. When a controlling young man isolates a woman from her friends, she becomes even more dependent on him for support, because she feels as if she has no one else in the whole wide world.

Julie and Jim were 16 when they first "hooked up" (became sexually involved) at a party. Jim was a star athlete in their high school. Both had experimented sexually before, but neither had been in an ongoing relationship.

After the party, Jim insisted that Julie hang out with him whenever he wasn't at practice. If her cell phone rang when they were together, Jim answered it himself, saying, "She's busy." He hung all over her at school, kissing her up against the lockers between classes, holding her on his lap in the cafeteria, and making out with her behind the bleachers when they skipped class together and snuck out. Jim told Julie her friends were "annoying," and she broke off contact with them. When he carried his control too far and Julie became angry with him, Jim bought her presents and took her out to dinner.

While Jim was away at football camp for a week, Julie gathered the courage to break up with him. Upon his return, Jim threatened to kill Julie and any boy who so much as looked at her. He waited for her after school every day, sometimes angry, sometimes romantic and kind. Soon they were a couple again.

If a teenager who is being controlled feels obligated to keep the relationship secret from her parents and other adults, a rift grows between her and those who might have been able to support her. She feels alone in trying to manage a relationship that is really too much for her.

Many teen relationships are marked by extreme jealousy. A male partner may become hostile or abusive if he sees or hears that his girlfriend (or ex-girlfriend) has spoken to other guys. He may enlist his own network of friends—and sometimes even her friends—to keep track of her movements. At the same time, he may brag to others about cheating on her.

A teen girl can also be extremely jealous and may call or text her boyfriend constantly, to check on his whereabouts. A girl may even physically strike out against her boyfriend (or another girl) if she suspects he has been "cheating." However, research shows that boys are more apt to feel amused or annoyed than seriously threatened if their girlfriend is excessively jealous, even if she physically assaults him.[5] Also, where the girlfriend is jealous and chooses to behave violently, she may be more likely to attack the other girl in question rather than her boyfriend, assessing that the other girl will be a less dangerous target.

Often a controlling young man will show possession of his girlfriend by touching her constantly, whenever they are together in public. He might hold her by the hand or have his arm around her, always, even at school or in front of her parents. Or he might hold her from behind and rub himself against her, with his hands wrapped tightly around her waist. He might insist on long tongue kisses, in public, whether she wants this or not. Of course, some young women enjoy this physical closeness. But some submit unhappily, feeling that the physical closeness is about possession, not affection.

IMAGE MANAGEMENT

Teen girls who engage, or are rumored to engage, in sexual activities may face the highly negative term "slut," whereas boys who engage in similar activities are positively viewed as "players" or "ladies' men." This sexual double standard sometimes traps teen girls in unhealthy relationships.

Ross and Dana first met when Ross was in his senior year of high school and Dana was a junior. Ross invited Dana to the prom, flattering her and raising her status in her peer group. One evening a week before prom, Ross took Dana out to the park. Dana was both excited and nervous. It was the first time that she had been out alone with a boy. She lied to her parents about where she was going, knowing they did not want her to start dating until she was 18. On a dark bench, Ross kissed Dana. He then put his hand on her breast. Dana tried pushing his hand away but Ross insisted. At one point Dana tried standing up but Ross pulled her back onto the bench, telling her, "You're too good to get away." He moved her hand onto his erection and told her, "You have to help me out now. You did this to me." He unzipped his pants and made her kneel, pushing her to suck his penis. When he was done, Dana was crying and Ross comforted her, saying, "You're my girl now." Ross implied that as long as she was with him and no one else, he would keep the secret of what had happened between them. Ross assured Dana that she was going to like it more in the future.

When she returned home, Dana saw that Ross had publicly thanked her on social media "for the good time." Ross set the terms of the relationship, told Dana where she could and could not go, and continued to push her sexually.

Quite a few factors trapped Dana in this relationship, including difficulties speaking with her parents and Ross's use of social and sexual pressure. She also felt trapped by fears about her reputation. If she had refused to be Ross's girlfriend, she reasoned, she would be considered "loose" for having had sexual contact with him.

Relationships among teens tend to be brief. Aware of this, some teens try to get as much benefit as possible from a relationship. Having a girlfriend, especially one who is considered "hot," raises a boy's social status. Having a girlfriend also helps a young man "prove" that he is not gay, to himself and others.

PHYSICAL ABUSE AND DOMINATION

Having recently grown through puberty, some adolescent males use their size to assert power over their teen partners. Often they present this as "play" but then take it further than the partner wants. A teenager might tickle his girlfriend or wrestle with her, continuing to roughhouse even when she asks him to stop and is clearly distressed. He may restrain her by twisting her arm up behind her back, holding her down, or grabbing her wrists, and then mock her if she becomes upset, saying he's "just messing with" her. A controlling young man might hit or slap his girlfriend, even in public, and define his actions as "just playing," criticizing her for being "no fun." If they go swimming, a young man might throw his girlfriend into the water or even dunk her and hold her under, gasping for air. Teenagers often flirt and establish physical closeness through play fighting. However, if one person does not desire the actions or experiences them as frightening, then it is not play but abuse.

A controlling boy does not always present these efforts to dominate physically as mere games. He might grab, push, slap, pinch, restrain, and even bite his girlfriend as a threat or punishment, or just to show "who's boss." The physical violence often begins when a girl refuses to engage in a particular sex act. Once the violence has begun, it may become a routine part of the relationship.

Like adult men, teen males often intimidate their partners physically through indirect violence. When they punch or kick walls, smash things, drive too fast, threaten physical violence, or fight with other boys, they are clearly conveying their violent tendencies.

Some teen boys let others know that when they are provoked they might "lose it" and be unable to control their words or actions. By the time they reach adulthood, men are usually expected to be able to "keep it together." But a self-proclaimed total loss of control may even be a point of pride for a young man and a threat to his partner.

DRINKING AND DRUGS

Those teenagers who use alcohol often binge, taking in a large amount in a short time. For teens, drinking alcohol is frequently seen as a path to getting drunk fast rather than as a social event to be savored. With disinhibition as the goal, it is unsurprising that many teens engage in bad behaviors in their drunken state that they would not allow themselves to engage in when sober.

Rui, 17, drank as many beers as he could get his hands on every Friday and Saturday night, usually at parties at friends' houses. When drinking, he would demand that his girlfriend, Hina, 16, stay within his sight at all times. He even insisted that she signal him when she was going to use the bathroom. He sometimes made her sit on his lap. He would make sexualized comments about her in front of their friends and would rub her thigh in a way that made her uncomfortable. Hina usually did not drink at these parties, and she would drive Rui home afterward. Once, on the drive home, Hina told Rui how unhappy she was with the way he had treated her at the party. He started shouting and grabbed the wheel. Hina felt in danger. When he was not drinking, Rui could act a little bossy at times, but Hina felt generally safe with him. Hina tried to drive other young people home after parties, in addition to Rui, so she would not have to be in the car alone with him when he had been drinking.

Many teen men press women to drink so they will accept sexual acts that they otherwise would reject. Sometimes these pressures can be quite deliberate and even organized. A group of young men might decide to play drinking games together with their girlfriends, so they can later force themselves on them. Having sex with someone who is not conscious or who is unable to give meaningful consent because of intoxication is rape and is a crime. Some young men deliberately press young women to drink and get high, encouraging them to "have another toke" or "just one more shot," knowing the girl's ability to protect herself may be weakened. This is a deliberate effort to "get them messed up" (incapacitate them).

Drugs can work similarly to alcohol, reducing the victimizer's inhibitions and making the victim more vulnerable. Some controlling teens become paranoid and extremely jealous when they have been smoking pot.

SEXUAL PRESSURE

Many young women face routine sexual pressure from their boyfriends and even from boys and men whom they do not know well. Young men who have managed to get close to a young woman may plead for more, saying that everyone is doing it, that she has led him on, and that he has certain needs. Also, teen boys often manipulate girls' ideas of love, with a version of "If you really loved me, you would . . . " Exposed to a lifetime of romantic stories about true love, teen girls may succumb to sexual coercion packaged as a declaration of love.

Typically, girls are seen as the gatekeepers of sexual activity, expected to put up some kind of resistance so they will not be labeled "sluts." At the same time, girls are expected to be popular and please boys, making it difficult for them to shout "rape," try to defend themselves physically, or refuse sexual advances clearly and explicitly. Perhaps because of their inexperience or a sense of entitlement, teen boys often pressure or force girls into sexual acts that are beyond the girls' comfort zone—acts that the girls have tried to refuse. Young men who are afraid of rejection often "take" rather than request sexual contact.

Sexual pressure within a controlling teen relationship can consist of pressing a partner to engage in sexual acts she does not want, or at times when she does not want them. Or a boy might refuse to practice safer sex. Another sign of coercive control is a young man pursuing only his own pleasure and disregarding his partner's pleasure. The very continuance of a sexual relationship may also be coerced, as girls try to break away and are harassed, followed, and assaulted until they give in.

> Facing frequent sexual pressures, teenage girls often give in rather than openly resist.

If a boy abandons his sexual pressure at a given moment but then storms off and insults his girlfriend or threatens to "find someone else who'll do it," the teenage girl learns she must meet his demands or risk losing the relationship. If he is somewhat older, he might induce her to go further than she wants sexually by accusing her of being immature and implying that he will look for satisfaction elsewhere if she does not comply. Sometimes teens feel pressured by their peer group to overstep their sexual boundaries or risk being labeled "uptight," "lame," or a "cocktease." And unfortunately, some controlling young men induce real fear in their partners, letting them know that refusing sex is not an option, so they had better comply if they don't want to be forced.

Girls commonly communicate their refusal by frowning, pushing away the boy's hands, or trying to leave the situation. Some teenage girls speak timidly, as if they are asking a question, and might say, "I'm not sure I want to do that" rather than clearly saying "stop." Many young men believe they are expected to push young women beyond their limits to achieve their own sexual satisfaction. And so some young men feel entitled to ignore a girl's direct or indirect refusal. After an unwanted sexual encounter, a boy may claim there was a misunderstanding and that he thought she really wanted it. In criminal rape trials, defendants frequently use the word "consensual" to justify their actions.

Some teen boys create a subculture that supports the sexual assault and coercion of girls. Boys sometimes place bets on how long it will take to lure a particular girl into bed, or they have contests to see how many girls they can seduce in a given period of time. In one school, the senior boys competed with each other to see how many of the sophomore girls they could "get." They deliberately targeted sophomores rather than freshman girls because they knew the statutory rape laws in their state did not cover relationships with only a two-year difference in age.

CELL PHONES AND COMPUTERS

Technology presents teenagers with new opportunities for coercive control. Most teens today use cell phones and computers regularly. This provides fertile ground for cyberstalking, harassing, and bullying (see also the section "Stalking and Monitoring," pages 30–32). Some abusive teens will almost constantly text, call, or instant message their partners. If the abuser cannot detect his girlfriend's whereabouts through technology, he may track her down in person or by texting her friends. Technology allows an abuser's reach to be extended even into his victim's parents' house, where he may insist on speaking with her, texting her, or chatting with her for hours on end. Not infrequently, parents think their adolescent children are asleep while the teens are actually busy chatting or texting their friends or romantic partners.

Twitter, Snapchat, Instagram, AskFM, and similar sites can all be used to threaten, express ownership over, or punish a partner or ex-partner. These communications can be hard to document and extremely frightening, as when a boyfriend sends a picture of a bloody knife over Snapchat to his ex-girlfriend and the image is set to dissolve in a few seconds.

Teen boys often keep "nudies" (naked photos) of their girlfriends and ex-girlfriends on their phones. When angry with a girlfriend or after they've broken up, it is not unusual for boys to trade these photos with their friends. In many high schools, pictures of naked girls circulate for years as they are traded among boys of various grades. Circulating a picture of a naked person under 18 is a serious crime. Teenagers (as well as adults) would be well advised to *never* allow naked pictures of themselves to be taken.

Some adult abusers use the Internet to meet and seduce minors. These adults usually are not entirely unknown to the teenager—they may be from the neighborhood, from school or church, or may be related to a friend. If these relationships persist over time, they can be extremely controlling.

> Sending or receiving a photo or video of a naked person under 18 is a serious crime. Teenagers (as well as adults) would be well advised to *never* allow naked pictures of themselves to be taken.

TEENS WITH OLDER PARTNERS

Some teens think they can learn from an older, more experienced partner, and through the partner gain entrance into an exciting, different social world. Teenagers may be impressed with some of the rewards of dating an older person, such as access to alcohol, drugs, and a car. Some teens also expect an older partner to be more mature and respectful.

However, it is rare for a teen partner to have equal power in a relationship where there is a great difference in age. The older person usually makes the decisions, and the younger person's ideas and opinions are apt to be brushed aside. Often, the younger partner has to ask permission to do things, alone or with friends or family.

Laverne was 16 when she met 28-year-old Dennis at the beach. Dennis spoke with Laverne politely and told her she had "killer eyes." He bought Laverne and her friend an ice cream. Laverne refused to give Dennis her phone number, but she told him how to contact her online. They began a frequent online correspondence and soon began texting. Two weeks later, Dennis picked up Laverne at school. When she entered his car, Dennis handed Laverne flowers. He took her out to dinner. This was her first "real date." At the end of the meal, Dennis told Laverne he was taking her to his apartment to meet his dog. Laverne told Dennis that she needed to get home and would rather meet the dog another time, but Dennis insisted. He said it would not take long. Laverne knew she was probably going to be pushed into sex, and she wanted to avoid this. But she also felt an obligation to be nice to Dennis, since he had been so generous with her.

Thus began their routine. Dennis picked up Laverne every couple of days after school and took her back to his apartment for sex. Dennis gave Laverne access to alcohol and bought her clothing and jewelry. He styled himself as her sexual teacher and punished her when he said she had misbehaved. He persuaded Laverne to enact scenes from porn movies at his house.

Laverne did not always want to go with Dennis after school. But if she saw his car parked outside, she felt compelled to get in, even if she felt she should be home studying for exams or if she'd rather be with her friends. Laverne became secretive and moody. She felt that Dennis had a certain power over her that she did not understand and did not know how to break. She was too intimidated to speak about it with others.

PREGNANT AND MOTHERING TEENS

When their partners get pregnant, men often increase their control. This may be especially true with pregnant teens. The father-to-be expects the young mother to stay home and rest for the benefit of their child while he continues to live a fuller life. Once the baby is born and is more mobile, some teen mothers want to assert themselves, move out into the world again, and "get on with" their lives. At this point conflict may erupt if the young man has become used to her staying at home.

Whether the father is an older man or a teenager himself, he might insist that the teen mother be responsible for all the child-care, while he remains free to continue school, work, and social activities. He tells the girl to "act like a mother" while he enjoys his freedom.

Other men who impregnate young women simply walk away and pretend the baby has nothing to do with them. Teen mothers who raise their children alone or with their own relatives, without the father's involvement, face many challenges. But at least they will not be subject to the control or abuse of the baby's father.

Teen mothers are stereotyped as irresponsible and promiscuous and as a public health problem. To avoid the additional stigma of being a *single* teen mom, many teenage girls struggle hard to maintain relationships with their child's father, even if that man is abusive or controlling. Staying with him may seem better than "becoming a statistic." Teen mothers who have been rejected by their families, who are isolated, and who don't access formal support services may be especially likely to maintain a relationship with the child's father, even at enormous cost to themselves. Teen mothers often lose contact with their friends, either because of their partners' control or because of their changed life circumstances. Participating in programs with other young mothers often helps them reduce their isolation and regain their self-confidence.

Social welfare programs often tout the virtues of involving young fathers in the lives of their children. While a father's participation is generally positive, a father who acts in a violent or controlling manner may pose more of a risk than a benefit to his child and to his child's mother. A controlling or abusive man should undergo a batterer intervention program before he is allowed to maintain contact with children he has fathered with a teen mother. Support programs must pay attention to

> A father who acts in a violent or controlling manner may pose more of a risk than a benefit to his child and to his child's mother.

the welfare of the young mothers, who are also minors in need of protection, as well as the welfare of their babies.

LGBT TEENS

Many LGBT teens have a hard time in high school and among their peers. They may be teased mercilessly at school. If they hide their sexual orientation or gender identity, then they live in perpetual fear of being "outed." Threatening to "out" a teen can serve as a powerful means of control for a partner or ex-partner. Depending on their location and their family's belief, a teen who is forcibly outed may be kicked out of their home or forced into abusive "reparative therapy."

Teens who have a tense relationship with their parents, or who have been forced to leave home because of their sexual orientation or gender identity, may find that an older partner offers benefits that a similar-age partner can't give them, such as a place to live and financial support. If they depend on their partners for these basic necessities, the teens will have more difficulty breaking off a problematic relationship.

LGBT teens may have difficulty meeting partners their own age. Therefore, they may fall prey more easily to adults looking for a relationship with a younger person. They may also have extra difficulty leaving a controlling relationship, believing it will be hard to find a new partner.

YOUNG PEOPLE HELPING EACH OTHER

If you are concerned about someone you know, the most important thing you can do is stay connected. Stay in touch with the person who is being controlled or abused. Invite that person out for walks, to events, or to your house. Make sure she understands that she still has friends and is not alone. Try to counteract the negative messages her boyfriend may be giving her. Ask her about the positive and negative aspects of her relationship. Ask her about her fears. Gently share your impressions, being sure not to sound judgmental. Avoid telling her what to do. Share this book with her. Help her check out websites on controlling and abusive relationships (see Chapter 11).

Carol and Shawn, who were both 16-year-old sophomores in high school, had been going out for a year. They mostly spent time alone with each other. Carol quit track and band. Her schoolwork slipped. She grew skinny, which first caused admiration, then alarm among her parents and friends. She seemed to lose interest in everything except being with Shawn. Both families approved of the relationship. Carol's parents thought Shawn was supportive of her daughter and even took him on a family vacation. Increasingly isolated, Carol made a couple of halfhearted suicidal gestures, once swallowing a handful of pills, and the next time scratching her wrist with a scissors.

Although they felt Carol had pushed them away, several of her friends from elementary and middle school grew concerned and decided to reach out to Carol. They sat with her in the cafeteria, ignoring Shawn's critical stares. They invited her to their houses. They told her, again and again, how much they liked her and that they had missed her. They shared food with her and noticed that as she put on a few pounds, she began to cheer up. They pushed her to try out for the school musical. She landed a big part and spent hours away from Shawn, at rehearsals.

After a few months, Carol seemed stronger. She realized that Shawn was holding her back from people and activities that she enjoyed. She broke up with him and ignored his requests to get back together. Her circle of friends played an important role in helping her regain her confidence and reclaim her life.

If you are going to help your friend, you must not spread gossip about her or about her relationship. Listen to her well and ask how you can help.

If possible, find a trustworthy adult with whom you can share your concerns. This might be a parent, school counselor, teacher, coach, or school nurse. Consider taking your friend to a domestic violence agency to meet with an advocate. Remember, if you discuss a minor who has been abused or who is at risk for being abused, or who is suicidal, that adult may have to alert authorities. Sometimes teenagers think the most important thing they can do is keep their friends' secrets from adults. While keeping confidences certainly is valuable, it is crucial for friends to keep each other safe.

FOR ADULTS WHO CARE ABOUT TEENS

Even more than adults, teenagers who are caught in a web of coercive control need the support of other people to help them break free. Teenagers do not have the experience, knowledge, confidence, or legal status to assert themselves completely. Unfortunately, teenagers frequently seek advice only from their peers, who may not be able to offer meaningful help. Adults who want to be a resource for teens must show themselves to be trustworthy. The adults must listen well and offer support before they jump in with advice.

> Listen well and offer support before you jump in with advice.

It is easy for adults to grow impatient when working with a teenager caught in an abusive or controlling relationship. We may wonder why the young person cannot seem to see the destructive effects of the relationship. We rush the teen to "hurry up and break up!" This is not always easy. We must remember how deeply most adolescents experience their feelings. They may feel loved for the first time, and doubt they will ever be loved again. They may believe the myth of *Beauty and the Beast* and other legends that their own pure, undying love will transform a difficult man into a prince. The relationship may give the teenager status or other benefits that are difficult for adults to appreciate.

Adults must be mindful of other forces that might keep a couple together. For example, a young woman may suspect that she is pregnant, or she may have moved out of her home or dropped out of school to live with her boyfriend. She may have been threatened with physical violence or her boyfriend's suicide if she breaks off the relationship. He may possess sexual photos or videos of her, or information about her, which he has threatened to release if she stops seeing him. She may have lost all her friends as she became more entwined with her abuser.

What, then, can a caring adult do to help a teenager caught in a relationship of coercive control? We can ask respectful questions. We can provide information, including this book and other materials and websites referenced in the Resources at the end of this book. We can accompany a controlled teen to a domestic violence agency, but then we should allow the young person to speak with an advocate alone. Domestic violence agencies can be very helpful to a teen who is caught in a controlling relationship.

For those teens still in school, educational campaigns that are directed to all students about healthy relationships will reach those who need them most. For maximum effectiveness, educators should be sure to involve students in designing and implementing these efforts.

Information on healthy relationships can be inserted into health or psychology classes, or into group sessions led by school counselors. Discussion groups about relationships, created for girls and boys, separately, can also be informative and empowering. Training in assertiveness, conflict resolution, and mediation all teach teens how to communicate with other people sensibly. Schoolwide training can reduce harassment as well as bullying. All teens should be taught about the legal penalties for cyberharassment and for circulating pictures of naked minors by phone or computer.

For LGBT teens, gay–straight alliances can be a lifesaver. So can adults who let others know they are comfortable speaking about LGBT issues. LGBT teens who find ways to meet potential partners their own age are less likely to fall victim to adult abusers.

Teens who are no longer in school need to be addressed where they spend time—on the Internet, at pizza parlors, and in malls. Teens who are in foster care, detention centers, or residential facilities need special outreach where they live. Doctor's offices and various public places can have discreet brochures available.

Adults who work with teens should become familiar with the various signs of coercive control. They should also educate teens about sexual consent, specifically, and healthy relationships in general. Teens often respond well to the following description of what is necessary for true consent in a relationship:

- **H**onesty
- **E**quity
- **R**espect and
- **S**afety

The initials spell HERS but it must be clear that—for heterosexual couples—the responsibility is HIS, too.[6]

Teens who are controlled by their partners often lose their freedom, their self-esteem, and opportunities for personal growth. All of this book should be helpful to them, even though some of the examples focus more on adults.

PART IV

Ending Coercive Control

These final chapters are for people who are being victim-ized and people who know someone personally or pro-fessionally who is being victimized. Chapter 7 is designed to help people assess their relationship for signs of coercive control and for danger. This section will also help you think about the many things you do to cope. Chapter 8 is for peo-ple who decide to stay in their relationship, for the short or long term. This chapter suggests ways to improve the rela-tionship so it will be safer and less restrictive. As you try these steps, you will be able to see whether an improved relationship is likely or even possible. Chapter 9 is for peo-ple who decide to leave their relationship or whose relation-ship has recently ended. This chapter discusses improving safety when leaving. Chapter 10 describes the path toward recovery.

Some women stay in a controlling relationship, waiting for it to improve, waiting for those moments of happiness with their partner, waiting for the children to grow up, or waiting for their partner to die. These waits can go on for years or decades. Only you can know whether the waiting is good for you and good for your children.

Are You Being Victimized?

If you wonder whether you are being victimized in a relationship of coercive control, this chapter will help you assess your situation. Your partner has probably told you that you are the problem, and you may wonder whether it is true. This chapter will help you get a realistic picture of those areas of your relationship that trouble you. This assessment process can help you see connections among experiences you have been through, but it may be painful. Please make sure you have support.

ASSESSING THE RELATIONSHIP

Let's assume you have some concerns about the quality or health of your relationship. Try to be hopeful about the possibility of freedom, whether that freedom takes the form of improving or ending the relationship.

> Be hopeful about the possibility of regaining your freedom and sense of self, whether this takes the form of improving or ending the relationship.

This section offers new ways to think about your relationship. It will help you reach a decision about whether you want to remain in the relationship and try to change it or end it completely. Below you will find a series of questions about some of the controlling behaviors you might be facing and some of the steps you have taken to cope with them. Take your time looking them over. Sit down with this book in a safe place and mark the answers. Feel free to make notes to yourself in the margins, including words that will remind you of specific events. Add items to the list in each section. If you are currently in a controlling relationship, make sure you keep the book in a safe place.

You might be surprised to recognize some familiar behaviors on the list that indicate coercive control. These might be actions that you are accustomed to, that just feel like "the way it is." People who are being victimized and then read this list sometimes begin to see their relationships in a new light and think about events quite differently. Other items on the list may seem quite extreme to you, and you may be relieved to realize that you do not face them.

There is no one right way to use this list. Unfortunately, you cannot simply add up the items, arrive at a total, and say to yourself, "My relationship is okay" or "My relationship is controlling and I have to change it" or "I must end this relationship." Coercive control varies widely from one relationship to another. These decisions are too individual for that kind of numerical process.

Not all the questions on this list are created equal. That is, responding "sometimes" to one question, such as "Does he threaten to kill you?" or "Does he try to keep you away from other people?" may be reason enough for you to end your relationship today. Responding "sometimes" to a question about whether he tries to control what you eat or how you spend money may not. Or it may. Only you can decide what is a valid reason to end the relationship.

Controlling Relationship Assessment*

Instructions: Please circle the word below that best answers each question. Skip questions that are not applicable.

Assessing Isolation

In general, does your partner try to keep you away from other people?

No   Yes

Does your partner *make demands* regarding your:

• Leaving the house?	NEVER	SOMETIMES	OFTEN/ALWAYS
• Telephone conversations?	NEVER	SOMETIMES	OFTEN/ALWAYS
• E-mail?	NEVER	SOMETIMES	OFTEN/ALWAYS
• Social media?	NEVER	SOMETIMES	OFTEN/ALWAYS
• Letters or other mail?	NEVER	SOMETIMES	OFTEN/ALWAYS
• Spending time with other people?	NEVER	SOMETIMES	OFTEN/ALWAYS
• Friendships?	NEVER	SOMETIMES	OFTEN/ALWAYS
• Relationships with your parents, brother or sister, or other family?	NEVER	SOMETIMES	OFTEN/ALWAYS
• Doing hobbies or activities with others?	NEVER	SOMETIMES	OFTEN/ALWAYS
• Joining organizations?	NEVER	SOMETIMES	OFTEN/ALWAYS

List other ways your partner *tries to keep you from contact with other people*:

• _____

• _____

• _____

---

*Adapted with permission from the authors from Dutton, M. A., Goodman, L., and Schmidt, R. J. (2006). *Development and validation of a coercive control measure for intimate partner violence: Final technical report*. Washington, DC: U.S. Department of Justice. Purchasers of this book can download and print this questionnaire in a larger format from *www.guilford.com/fontes3-forms*.

Personal Activities

In general, does your partner try to control your personal activities?

No   Yes

Does your partner *make demands* regarding your:

• Sleeping	NEVER	SOMETIMES	OFTEN/ALWAYS
• Wearing certain clothes?	NEVER	SOMETIMES	OFTEN/ALWAYS
• Using television, radio, or the Internet?	NEVER	SOMETIMES	OFTEN/ALWAYS
• Pursuing hobbies or other interests?	NEVER	SOMETIMES	OFTEN/ALWAYS
• Reading certain things?	NEVER	SOMETIMES	OFTEN/ALWAYS
• Taking care of the house?	NEVER	SOMETIMES	OFTEN/ALWAYS
• Taking care of your appearance (makeup, grooming)?	NEVER	SOMETIMES	OFTEN/ALWAYS

List other ways your partner *tries to control your personal activities*:

- _____
- _____
- _____

Resources: Education, Work, and Money

In general, does your partner try to control your education, work, or money?   No   Yes

Does your partner *make demands* regarding your:

• Work activities?	NEVER	SOMETIMES	OFTEN/ALWAYS
• Career or job path?	NEVER	SOMETIMES	OFTEN/ALWAYS
• Spending money?	NEVER	SOMETIMES	OFTEN/ALWAYS
• Credit or credit history?	NEVER	SOMETIMES	OFTEN/ALWAYS
• Going to school/learning new skills?	NEVER	SOMETIMES	OFTEN/ALWAYS
• Accessing transportation (car, truck, or money for public transportation)?	NEVER	SOMETIMES	OFTEN/ALWAYS

List other ways your partner *tries to control your education, work, or money*:

- _____
- _____
- _____

Health and Body

In general, does your partner try to control aspects of your health or body?

No   Yes

Does your partner *make demands* regarding your:

• Eating or weight?	NEVER	SOMETIMES	OFTEN/ALWAYS
• Sleeping?	NEVER	SOMETIMES	OFTEN/ALWAYS
• Bathing or using the bathroom?	NEVER	SOMETIMES	OFTEN/ALWAYS

Does your partner *block* you from:

• Taking prescription drugs that you need?	NEVER	SOMETIMES	OFTEN/ALWAYS
• Going for medical care?	NEVER	SOMETIMES	OFTEN/ALWAYS
• Doing exercise?	NEVER	SOMETIMES	OFTEN/ALWAYS

Does your partner *push* you to:

• Use street drugs?	NEVER	SOMETIMES	OFTEN/ALWAYS
• Use prescription drugs for nonmedical reasons?	NEVER	SOMETIMES	OFTEN/ALWAYS
• Drink alcohol or drink more alcohol than you want?	NEVER	SOMETIMES	OFTEN/ALWAYS
• Get tattoos or piercings?	NEVER	SOMETIMES	OFTEN/ALWAYS
• Get breast implants, liposuction, a facelift, or other cosmetic surgery?	NEVER	SOMETIMES	OFTEN/ALWAYS
• Stop seeing a psychotherapist or counselor?	NEVER	SOMETIMES	OFTEN/ALWAYS

List other ways your partner *makes demands regarding your body or health*:

* _____
* _____
* _____

Intimacy

In general, does your partner try to control your intimate relationship?

No   Yes

Does your partner *make demands* regarding:

• Having sex?	NEVER	SOMETIMES	OFTEN/ALWAYS
• Avoiding the use of condoms or other birth control?	NEVER	SOMETIMES	OFTEN/ALWAYS
• Doing certain sexual behaviors?	NEVER	SOMETIMES	OFTEN/ALWAYS
• Taking sexual pictures or videos?	NEVER	SOMETIMES	OFTEN/ALWAYS

Does your partner *block* your efforts to:

• Separate or leave the relationship?	NEVER	SOMETIMES	OFTEN/ALWAYS
• Speak about things that matter to you?	NEVER	SOMETIMES	OFTEN/ALWAYS

List other ways your partner *tries to control your intimate relationship*:

* _____
* _____
* _____

Authorities

In general, does your partner try to control your relationship with authorities?   No   Yes

Does your partner *make demands* regarding:

• Talking to the police or a lawyer?	NEVER	SOMETIMES	OFTEN/ALWAYS
• Talking to a landlord or housing authority?	NEVER	SOMETIMES	OFTEN/ALWAYS

Does your partner fail to help you improve your citizenship status? (Leave blank if not applicable.)

No   Yes

Does your partner push you to do things that are against the law (commit crimes)?

No   Yes

List other ways your partner *interferes with your relationship with authorities*:

- _____
- _____
- _____

Children

(skip this section if there are no children involved in your relationship)

In general, does your partner try to control your relationship with your children?

No   Yes

Does your partner *interfere* with your:

• Taking care of the children?	NEVER	SOMETIMES	OFTEN/ALWAYS
• Setting rules for or disciplining the children?	NEVER	SOMETIMES	OFTEN/ALWAYS
• Making everyday decisions about the children?	NEVER	SOMETIMES	OFTEN/ALWAYS
• Making important decisions about the children?	NEVER	SOMETIMES	OFTEN/ALWAYS
• Talking to child protection authorities?	NEVER	SOMETIMES	OFTEN/ALWAYS

Does your partner:

• Turn your children against you?	NEVER	SOMETIMES	OFTEN/ALWAYS
• Threaten to or call social services to say you are neglecting or abusing the children when you are not?	NEVER	SOMETIMES	OFTEN/ALWAYS

- Threaten to get custody of the   NEVER   SOMETIMES   OFTEN/ALWAYS
  children if you try to leave the
  relationship?

- Mistreat the children and blame it   NEVER   SOMETIMES   OFTEN/ALWAYS
  on your parenting problems?

List other ways your partner *interferes with your relationship with your children*:

- _____

- _____

- _____

Monitoring

In general, does your partner try to find out what you have done and where you have been?   No   Yes

Does your partner:

- Check, read, or destroy your mail?   NEVER   SOMETIMES   OFTEN/ALWAYS

- Check, read, or block your e-mail?   NEVER   SOMETIMES   OFTEN/ALWAYS

- Keep track of your telephone or   NEVER   SOMETIMES   OFTEN/ALWAYS
  cell phone use?

- Keep track of your computer use?   NEVER   SOMETIMES   OFTEN/ALWAYS

- Call you on the phone to check on   NEVER   SOMETIMES   OFTEN/ALWAYS
  you?

- Tell you to carry a cell phone so he NEVER   SOMETIMES   OFTEN/ALWAYS
  (or she) can check on you?

- Monitor your online activities?   NEVER   SOMETIMES   OFTEN/ALWAYS

- Check your clothing, purse, or   NEVER   SOMETIMES   OFTEN/ALWAYS
  home for signs that you have "done
  something wrong"?

- Check up on you through your   NEVER   SOMETIMES   OFTEN/ALWAYS
  receipts, checkbook, or bank
  statements?

- Check the car (odometer, where   NEVER   SOMETIMES   OFTEN/ALWAYS
  parked, looking for things)? (Leave
  blank if not applicable.)

- Ask you detailed questions about   NEVER   SOMETIMES   OFTEN/ALWAYS
  your activities?

- Use an audio or video recorder   NEVER   SOMETIMES   OFTEN/ALWAYS
  with you against your will?

- Spy on you, follow you, or stalk   NEVER   SOMETIMES   OFTEN/ALWAYS
  you?

- Ask other people about where you   NEVER   SOMETIMES   OFTEN/ALWAYS
  have been or what you have done?

- Get other people to keep track of   NEVER   SOMETIMES   OFTEN/ALWAYS
  you?

List other ways your partner *stalks or monitors you*:

- _____

- _____

- _____

Making You Feel Afraid

In general, does your partner make you feel afraid *to get you to do what he wants*?   No   Yes

Does your partner *make you feel afraid* by doing any of the following:

- Swearing, name-calling, and   NEVER   SOMETIMES   OFTEN/ALWAYS
  insulting?

- Getting in your face/standing too   NEVER   SOMETIMES   OFTEN/ALWAYS
  close?

- Throwing, kicking, or punching   NEVER   SOMETIMES   OFTEN/ALWAYS
  things?

- Slamming doors or stomping   NEVER   SOMETIMES   OFTEN/ALWAYS
  around?

- Grabbing or pushing you?   NEVER   SOMETIMES   OFTEN/ALWAYS

- Making you feel trapped in a room   NEVER   SOMETIMES   OFTEN/ALWAYS
  or pinned against a wall?

- Following you around?   NEVER   SOMETIMES   OFTEN/ALWAYS

- Refusing to speak with you for   NEVER   SOMETIMES   OFTEN/ALWAYS
  long periods of time?

- Leaving without telling you where   NEVER   SOMETIMES   OFTEN/ALWAYS
  he is going or for how long, to
  alarm you?

- Driving fast or recklessly while   NEVER   SOMETIMES   OFTEN/ALWAYS
  you or your children are in the car?

List other ways your partner *makes you feel afraid as a way to control you*:

- _____

- _____

- _____

Threatening Harm

In this section, please respond in terms of your partner's *threats*. In the next
section you can record things he has actually done.

In general, does your partner *threaten you to get you to do what he wants*?

No   Yes

To get you to do what he (or she) wants, has your partner *threatened* to:

- Reveal private information about   NEVER   SOMETIMES   OFTEN/ALWAYS
  you to others?

- Make you look bad in front of   NEVER   SOMETIMES   OFTEN/ALWAYS
  others?

- Share intimate personal photos   NEVER   SOMETIMES   OFTEN/ALWAYS
  of you or information about you
  electronically?

- Keep you from going where you   NEVER   SOMETIMES   OFTEN/ALWAYS
  want?

- Leave the relationship or get a   NEVER   SOMETIMES   OFTEN/ALWAYS
  divorce?

- Hurt you financially?   NEVER   SOMETIMES   OFTEN/ALWAYS

- Cause you legal trouble?   NEVER   SOMETIMES   OFTEN/ALWAYS

- Cause you to get in trouble at work   NEVER   SOMETIMES   OFTEN/ALWAYS
  or lose your job?

- Cause you to lose housing?   NEVER   SOMETIMES   OFTEN/ALWAYS

- Hurt you physically?   NEVER   SOMETIMES   OFTEN/ALWAYS

• Have sex with someone else?	NEVER	SOMETIMES	OFTEN/ALWAYS
• Force you to engage in unwanted sex acts?	NEVER	SOMETIMES	OFTEN/ALWAYS
• Damage or destroy something that belongs to you?	NEVER	SOMETIMES	OFTEN/ALWAYS
• Hurt or kill your pet or other animal?	NEVER	SOMETIMES	OFTEN/ALWAYS
• Take your children from you or harm your children?	NEVER	SOMETIMES	OFTEN/ALWAYS
• Kill himself?	NEVER	SOMETIMES	OFTEN/ALWAYS
• Kill you?	NEVER	SOMETIMES	OFTEN/ALWAYS

List other ways your partner has *threatened you to get you to do what he wants*:

• _____

• _____

• _____

Punishing or Harming You

In general, does your partner punish you or harm you?   No   Yes

Has your partner done any of the following things *as a punishment*?

• Said something mean, embarrassing, or degrading to you?	NEVER	SOMETIMES	OFTEN/ALWAYS
• Revealed private information about you to others?	NEVER	SOMETIMES	OFTEN/ALWAYS
• Kept you from going where you want?	NEVER	SOMETIMES	OFTEN/ALWAYS
• Had sex with someone else?	NEVER	SOMETIMES	OFTEN/ALWAYS
• Left the relationship or stormed out without explanation?	NEVER	SOMETIMES	OFTEN/ALWAYS
• Kept you out of your home?	NEVER	SOMETIMES	OFTEN/ALWAYS
• Hurt you financially?	NEVER	SOMETIMES	OFTEN/ALWAYS
• Caused you legal trouble?	NEVER	SOMETIMES	OFTEN/ALWAYS

• Caused you to get in trouble at work or lose your job?	NEVER	SOMETIMES	OFTEN/ALWAYS
• Caused you to lose housing?	NEVER	SOMETIMES	OFTEN/ALWAYS
• Damaged or destroyed something that belongs to you (on purpose)?	NEVER	SOMETIMES	OFTEN/ALWAYS
• Destroyed property of a friend or family member?	NEVER	SOMETIMES	OFTEN/ALWAYS
• Hurt or killed your pet or other animal?	NEVER	SOMETIMES	OFTEN/ALWAYS
• Kept you from your children or tried to take your children from you?	NEVER	SOMETIMES	OFTEN/ALWAYS
• Made you look bad in front of others?	NEVER	SOMETIMES	OFTEN/ALWAYS
• Attempted suicide or made suicidal gestures?	NEVER	SOMETIMES	OFTEN/ALWAYS
• Physically hurt your friend or family member?	NEVER	SOMETIMES	OFTEN/ALWAYS
• Hurt you physically without leaving a mark?	NEVER	SOMETIMES	OFTEN/ALWAYS
• Injured you physically (leaving a bruise, broken bone, or a sore area that lasted more than an hour, or made you bleed)?	NEVER	SOMETIMES	OFTEN/ALWAYS
• Choked, smothered, or tried to strangle you?	NEVER	SOMETIMES	OFTEN/ALWAYS
• Hurt you during sex or forced you to engage in unwanted sex acts?	NEVER	SOMETIMES	OFTEN/ALWAYS
• Caused you to fear for your life?	NEVER	SOMETIMES	OFTEN/ALWAYS
• Tried to kill you?	NEVER	SOMETIMES	OFTEN/ALWAYS

List other ways your partner has *punished or harmed you*:

• _____

• _____

• _____

The preceding list of controlling behaviors is not complete. You might have a few that you'd like to add. Many of the items on the list are against the law.

Examine your responses to the items above. Of the items that you marked "sometimes" or "often/always," which are the most upsetting to you? Which frighten you the most?

> • Do you have reason to think your partner will *continue doing* the behaviors? (Remember, past behavior is the best predictor of the future. Without some intense motivation, people don't usually change behaviors they have practiced for a long time—especially if these behaviors seem to be working for them.)
>
> • Do you have any reason to think your partner will engage in these behaviors *more severely or more often*?
>
> • Do you have any reason to think your partner could *stop doing* those behaviors that are most troubling to you? What would persuade him to stop?
>
> • What changes have you seen over time?

Discuss your answers to all the questions above with someone you can trust such as a therapist, an advocate, or a best friend. It is often better to speak with a professional than a friend, because with a friend you may be tempted to hide some of the problems. Also consider keeping a journal about these questions if you can store it in a safe place. If you feel overwhelmed by the questions, put them away for a few days or decide that you will think about them each day at a certain time while sitting or walking in a certain place. And when that time is over, pack them away in your mind like in a suitcase. Doing this helps many people avoid feeling overwhelmed.

Assessing Lethality: Risk of Death

Many people suffer greatly in relationships of coercive control, whether or not physical violence is present. Research shows that certain patterns increase the likelihood that a woman will be killed by her partner or former partner. Below are six questions related to serious physical danger. **Responding "yes" to any of these questions shows you are at greater risk that your intimate partner might try to kill you than people who can respond "no" to all of them.** (Unfortunately, responding "no" to the questions is not a guarantee of safety.) These questions refer to a partner or ex-partner[†]:

Has your partner ever used or threatened to use a gun, knife, or other weapon against you?	No	Yes
Has your partner ever tried or threatened to kill or injure you?	No	Yes
Has your partner choked, strangled, or smothered you?	No	Yes
Is your partner violently or constantly jealous?	No	Yes
Has your partner ever physically forced you to have sex?	No	Yes
Does your partner have access to a gun?	No	Yes

If you have answered "yes" to one or more of those questions, you are at higher risk than other women in controlling and abusive relationships. Consult with domestic violence advocates and the police to help assure your safety.

Assessing Your Coping Strategies

Even as they suffer from coercive control, most victims find ways to keep the peace and stay as safe and free as possible, given their partner. Think about everything you do on a regular basis to keep your wits about you despite the pressures of your relationship. Do

---

[†]Adapted from *http://justicewomen.com/tips_dv_assessment.html.*

you have safety zones where you can be yourself? Do you have routines or thoughts that keep you going? If you have children, think about everything you do to protect them and assure them a better future. Consider your strengths. Even if you are being victimized, you are much more than a victim. Here is a very short list of coping strategies; probably you do much more. Notice there is a new option here: "Want to do more." This is intended to help you note and remember some of the things you could do that might help you achieve greater freedom of movement and feel more like yourself again. Not all of these strategies will help you in the long run—some will help you feel better in the short run, while making life more difficult long-term.

- Do you stay in touch with friends? NEVER SOMETIMES OFTEN
  WANT TO DO MORE

- Do you stay in touch with family? NEVER SOMETIMES OFTEN
  WANT TO DO MORE

- Do you keep up hobbies? NEVER SOMETIMES OFTEN
  WANT TO DO MORE

- Do you belong to any organizations or clubs? NEVER SOMETIMES OFTEN
  WANT TO DO MORE

- Do you take some time for yourself each day? NEVER SOMETIMES OFTEN
  WANT TO DO MORE

- Do you take care of your health? NEVER SOMETIMES OFTEN
  WANT TO DO MORE

- Do you have short term goals for yourself? NEVER SOMETIMES OFTEN
  WANT TO DO MORE

- Do you have long term goals for yourself? NEVER SOMETIMES OFTEN
  WANT TO DO MORE

- Do you meditate or pray? NEVER SOMETIMES OFTEN
  WANT TO DO MORE

• Do you have a strategy to handle your partner's angry outbursts?	NEVER SOMETIMES OFTEN WANT TO DO MORE
• Do you try reasoning with your partner?	NEVER SOMETIMES OFTEN WANT TO DO MORE
• Do you use sex to help your partner calm down?	NEVER SOMETIMES OFTEN WANT TO DO MORE
• Do you bring or send your children to a safe place when it looks like your partner is getting angry?	NEVER SOMETIMES OFTEN WANT TO DO MORE
• Do you speak with a counselor, therapist, or advocate about what's going on?	NEVER SOMETIMES OFTEN WANT TO DO MORE
• Do you call the police when there are violent incidents?	NEVER SOMETIMES OFTEN WANT TO DO MORE
• Do you have a safety plan?	NEVER SOMETIMES OFTEN WANT TO DO MORE
• Do you use alcohol, drugs, or prescription medication to help you cope with your partner?	NEVER SOMETIMES OFTEN WANT TO DO LESS

List other *things you do to cope*:

* _____

* _____

* _____

Final Thoughts on Assessing Your Relationship

You may wonder why all the questions above focus on the bad parts of the relationship rather than the good ones. Many controlling people are experts at emphasizing the good parts of the relationship, possibly the financial security, the stable home for the children, the good sex, and that complicated four-letter word: LOVE. You are not being asked to review the positive parts of your relationship here because most people in controlling relationships are already well aware of them. And no matter how fine and enjoyable the good parts are, you need to ask yourself whether they are enough to make you tolerate feeling unfree. *Only you can decide.*

In couples, certainly, both people influence each other. People are not perfect. For example, one person yells when upset while another doesn't help with the housework. Sometimes couples become irritated with each other or accuse their partner of being "too bossy." Sometimes one person pushes the other to do something he or she would rather not do—to help out the other person or to help the family.

How can we tell the difference between ordinary relationship issues and harmful problems involving coercive control? First, we need to remember that coercive control exists on a spectrum. This ranges from relationships that are not at all controlling to those that are abusively controlling. People are comfortable at different spots on that spectrum. The difference between relationships of coercive control and other relationships may boil down to the following three words: isolation, fear, and punishment. People should not feel isolated or afraid in their intimate relationships. Members of a couple should not use threats or punishment to control each other. In your relationship, if one person feels afraid of, threatened by, or punished by the other—it is likely to be a relationship of coercive control.

REACHING A DECISION

What do you need in your life to feel like a complete and free human being? People subject to relationships of coercive control rarely ask themselves this question. They may have been told that this is a selfish question. It is an essential question. *Ask yourself this question several times a day. Identifying your needs will point you toward your goals.*

Also, think about your own opinions regarding the small and large things in life—from your favorite foods to politics to ideas for your own future. When in a relationship of coercive control, women often hear that their opinions are stupid. Their partners often respond angrily if they express their beliefs. In response, women sometimes begin to accept their partner's opinions as their own and lose a sense of their separate views. Recovering your own opinions and perspectives will help you feel like a more complete person, whatever decision you make regarding your relationship.

- What are your worst fears about staying in the relationship?
- What are your worst fears about ending it?
- Which are most likely?
- What can you change so you can achieve the best outcome—whichever path you choose?

These are all difficult but necessary questions. Again, talk them over with a professional counselor, advocate, or trusted friend. Consider writing in a journal about them if you can store it safely.

You may be at a crossroads where you are considering ending the relationship. If so, you are apt to feel some combination of fear, sadness, anger, and confusion. You probably feel quite alone. You may have hidden the problems in your relationship because you felt ashamed, because your partner asked you to, or because you didn't want people to think badly about you or your partner. If you hide parts of your relationship from your friends and family, this increases the likelihood that they will not grasp what you are going through.

You may fear that other people cannot understand your decisions. They may not understand why you stayed together or why you are thinking of breaking up. They may not know how excellent the good parts of the relationship are or once were. Most likely, they do not know about the bad parts either. If your partner is controlling but not physically violent, then it may be harder for you to figure out whether his behavior is abusive. You may be uncertain whether you would be better off living without him. Certainly, you may worry about money, children, housing, your safety, and a host of other issues if you decide to end the relationship. You may feel indebted to your partner.

You may believe you cannot live without your partner or that your partner cannot live without you. While breaking up a relationship can be excruciatingly painful, especially at first, the pain fades over time and new possibilities appear. You do not have to live in a relationship where you feel restricted or degraded, or where you tread carefully all the time in fear of angering your partner. If you have tried to make the relationship work and what you are going through is not acceptable, then maybe it is time to end the relationship.

Your partner may have persuaded you that he is the only person who could ever love you or want to be with you. He may have whittled down your self-esteem to make you believe that you will not love or be loved again if you end your relationship. You may fear that you will never find a love as intense or as deep. Of course, there are no guarantees about what the future holds. But someone who truly loves you would try to build you up, not tear you down. He would tell you how lovable you are, rather than making you feel bad about yourself. Even if your partner does not want to lose you, someone who truly loves you would not try to do you harm when you break things off. *If you decide to end the relationship, you are not doing something bad, even though it might feel bad. You have the right to make decisions about your own life, including your intimate relationship.*

If there are children involved, it is not good for them to see this coercive control relationship as a model of how people should treat each other. They should see their parents as free and fulfilled. They should see partners behave consistently in loving ways with each other.

Margaret decided rather suddenly to leave her husband. After years of tolerating control and verbal abuse, she glanced at her children's faces while her husband humiliated her at the breakfast table one day. "I left him for them," she said. "I was staying with him for the kids, but then I realized they were watching us closely and learning how to act from us. I wanted different models for them."

Consider the section "Protect Your Children" (pages 171–173).

8

Are You Staying?
Expecting Change?

People stay in controlling relationships for many reasons. If you are deciding whether to stay in a relationship, it can be hard to know if your decision is a "good" one. In a couple of years, will you look back on your decision and regret it? Unfortunately, no magic wand exists to point out the best path. But if you're caught in a controlling relationship, there are ways to improve your safety. And if your abuser says he wants to change, there are ways to assess whether he really is changing.

STAYING IN THE RELATIONSHIP

Maybe you have decided to stay in your relationship, for now at least, even though you believe you are being subject to coercive control. This section will give you some ideas about becoming a freer and safer person within that relationship. As you decide whether these ideas are possible in your situation, you may gain insight as to whether you want to leave or stay in

> Some relationships are "fixable"—the controlling partner makes real and lasting change. Most are not.

the long run. Some relationships are "fixable"—the controlling partner makes real and lasting change. Most are not.

The following tips can help you stay safe and retain your perspective on your life.

• **Make sure you stay connected to people beyond your relationship**, such as friends, neighbors, and family.

• **Join a group or organization** such as a chorus, book group, or parent–teacher organization. This will help you stay "in the world" and prevent isolation.

• **Seek the help of professionals** who are knowledgeable about these issues such as a domestic violence advocate, a counselor, or psychotherapist. Your friends may want to see you two stay together for their own reasons, or may grow weary of hearing the same stories again and again. Also, people who are being victimized often edit out parts of what they tell their friends, because they feel ashamed. Speaking openly with a professional can bring tremendous relief.

• **Straighten out your finances.** Sometimes controlling men have managed to place ownership of joint possessions—or even the woman's own possessions—under his name alone. If this has happened to you, and if it is safe, even if you are not planning to break up, get these situations corrected. Speak to a lawyer. Women's centers can usually recommend lawyers who are knowledgeable about how controlling men try to manipulate women's finances, and they can help you protect your rights. Some will work for women who have been abused without charging a fee.

• **Develop habits that regularly take you out of the home** such as taking out the trash, going for a walk, or buying a newspaper or pack of gum each day. This activity can be used as an excuse to leave if you have warning that abuse is likely to occur.

• **Store copies of important phone numbers and essential documents** in a safe place outside your home. These will give you a sense of security.

- **Make a list of your goals** and keep the list in a safe place. For instance, write down if you want to go back to school in a year, or visit your sister every two weeks, or begin to apply to jobs within a month, or go for a walk each day. Number your goals, starting with the small steps that seem easiest to accomplish. Put a star next to those that seem most essential. It is important for you to include your larger life goals as well as lesser ones, because you can achieve your dreams only if you identify them and then take baby steps toward making them come true. Discuss your goals with others. Commit to your goals. Imagine yourself achieving them. Plan for them. If it is safe to do so, discuss a goal with your partner and tell him you want his support. His response will provide you with valuable information. While his verbal support is welcome, it is even more important to see how he actually helps you achieve your goals. Or does he stand in your way?

- **Make a list of your limits**, too, and keep it in a safe place. For instance, write down if you refuse to be subjected to physical pain by your partner ever again. Or write down if you don't want to be blamed when you have done nothing wrong. You are the one who decides how much is too much. This is not your partner's decision, your child's decision, your religion's decision, or your family's decision. If it is safe, discuss your limits with your partner, one at a time. See how he responds. If he responds harshly, saying he feels you are telling him what he can and cannot do, this is a sign of his unwillingness to change. Also, he may obey "the letter of the law" by not slapping you, for instance, or not opening your mail, but still grab you harshly or look through your phone. Your list of limits is not a technical document. If your partner seems to want to "sneak in" mistreatment that is not covered, he is providing helpful information to you. This list is a declaration of your own worth. You have the right to live a life free of violence and control, even if your partner claims to love you.

> You are the one who decides how much is too much.

> You have the right to live a life free of violence and control, even if your partner claims to love you.

- **Set a time each week** to assess your progress toward your goals. Is the relationship moving in the right direction?

- **Consider seeking legal counsel** about finances and child custody, so you will know what you face if you do decide to leave at some point down the road.

- **Make a safety plan.** Safety plans, including items like those listed above, can help you stay safe in your relationship.

Quite a few of the suggestions above involve setting up "safety zones": places, relationships, and habits where you can feel free and like yourself.

As you look carefully at your relationship, you might feel a great deal of pain. Make sure you are not facing this alone. Seek the support of other people. Staying connected to other people will help you feel stronger as you think through the problems in your relationship.

IF A CONTROLLING PERSON WANTS TO CHANGE

A person who controls his partner benefits from this arrangement. Having a relationship with a woman who is afraid of him and who regularly puts his needs ahead of her own makes some men feel strong and loved. A controlling partner often believes that his power over his partner will keep her from leaving.

However, sometimes a controlling man genuinely wants to change. Maybe he regrets having physically or emotionally hurt his partner or children. Afraid of facing a jail sentence related to his abusive or controlling behaviors, maybe he wants to be a different kind of man. Maybe he has decided that he has lost too many relationships. Maybe he is tired of being angry, tired of feeling alone and misunderstood, and tired of monitoring another person. His own jealousy may exhaust him. He might remind himself of another person he never wanted to resemble—perhaps his father or stepfather. Maybe he is ready to change.

Following is a list of steps that an abuser should take if he is serious about changing. He needs to engage in every one that fits his situation; he cannot pick and choose. And he needs help for this process from someone other than his partner or ex-partner. Many men have tried unsuccessfully to change their habits alone. Seeking help will assure a better outcome.

The controlling person needs to:

- **Decide that he really wants to change.** Does he want to wake up a year from now caught in the same struggles, feeling the same feelings, hurting others in the same way? Only a deep determination to change will make him do the hard work that will be required of him.

- **Find his own motivation for changing.** Maybe his wife or girlfriend will leave the relationship regardless of what he does, or she has already left. He needs to decide to change for his own sake and for the sake of possible future relationships—not to keep her tied to him.

- **Stop blaming everyone else.** His controlling behaviors are not the fault of his wife or girlfriend, his parents or boss or society. He is making a choice every time he behaves in an abusive or controlling way. He needs to accept responsibility for his actions, even if his partner does something that makes him angry.

- **Join a batterer intervention program.** These groups are the right place for a controlling person, even one who has not physically assaulted his partner. Many of the same remedies apply if he has controlled his partner coercively. The most effective groups meet weekly and last at least six months. He needs to commit to going to every session and not dropping out. Many men who begin these groups are not strong enough to stick with them. He needs to decide not to quit—no matter how hard the going gets, and it will get tough. The facilitators and the other group members will help him understand the various ways he has been abusive and controlling in the distant and recent past. Becoming accountable is difficult, but many men report that it's a relief, too. In the group, he will also learn how to trust and speak more openly with other men. (An anger management program is not the right place for a man who uses coercive control with his partner. Anger management programs are too short and are geared toward men who explode or have "a short fuse" in general. They do not address the specifics of coercively controlling a partner.)

- **Accept that women (including his wife or girlfriend) are fully human**, with their own opinions, dreams, and desires apart from his. His partner's entire life should not revolve around him, and she should feel free to express her opinions.

- **Stop seeing himself as having a right to make all the decisions** even though he is a man and even if he earns all or most of the money.

- **Respect his partner's limits**—even if this is not what he wants. If she does not want to talk, if she does not want to listen, if she does not want to have sex—this is her right. When she says, "No," he needs to accept it without pushing her to bend to his will. She also has the right to leave the relationship if she chooses—as he does.

- **Respect his partner's independence.** She should be able to choose her friends. She deserves privacy. And she deserves to live free from insults, threats, fear, and punishment.

- **Let go of his terror about the relationship ending.** Some men believe they would rather die than give up a relationship with a particular woman—and they control her to try to keep her from leaving. Their feelings of attachment can be so intense—it does feel like a death to face separation. But it is not death. He can face separation, if this is his path, and survive. Life will be worth living. It's just going to hurt for a time.

- **Choose to act differently.** He needs to admit that he does have control over what he does and says. After all, even controlling men do not try to control everyone in their lives. Probably he just tries to control his partner and possibly any children in their lives. He must deny himself permission to act in controlling or abusive ways with the people who are close to him.

• **Redefine love** so it no longer serves as an excuse for jealous or controlling behavior. Love requires respect and kindness. Love does not pardon all.

• **Seek treatment for drugs or alcohol abuse or mental health issues if he needs it.** His controlling behaviors may lessen but are not apt to disappear if he resolves his depression, anxiety, trauma symptoms, or substance abuse problem. These are separate issues. However, he will not be able to change his controlling behavior unless he faces these other issues, too. Twelve-step groups such as Alcoholics Anonymous help many people.

Why would a controlling man try to give up his habits of coercive control? What's in it for him? Men who have stopped using coercive control find that both they themselves and their partners are happier and more fulfilled. Their relationships feel stronger and more genuine. Their children stop being afraid of them. Often they find they are able to enjoy better friendships as well—friendships where they can truly connect. After overcoming their coercive habits, many men feel more at peace with themselves. Change is difficult. But—for most controlling men—staying the same is also difficult. Generally, controlling men are not happy. (Consider the resources for controlling and abusive men listed at the end of this book, pages 203–207.)

> It is difficult for controlling men to change. But staying the same is also difficult.

How Do You Know If a Controlling or Abusive Person Has Changed?

It is easy for controlling men to promise to change. It is much more difficult for them to make a permanent change in their beliefs and actions.

Your partner may promise to change. Probably, you have heard such promises before. He may transform his behavior for a while based on sheer willpower. But deep and lasting change requires an extensive process over a long period of time.

If you do not live together or you have managed to move out or persuaded him to move out, do not move back in together until at least a year has passed in which you have seen consistent improvements. In that year, make sure that you have your autonomy and that he respects your decisions. Make sure he respects your need for time alone and with other people. If after a year you are still not sure you want to live with him, take more time.

If you move in with him again because he is leaving you no other options, you are already trapped.

Reuniting might make it harder to end the relationship down the road. You have no obligation to re-enter a relationship that makes you feel uncomfortable, even if there are children involved. If you return simply because you feel like he is leaving you no other options, you are already trapped.

Following are two lists: one of signs that your partner has *not* changed, despite his promises, and the other a list of signs that he has, indeed, changed. Read these from time to time as you assess your relationship.

Signs That a Controlling or Abusive Person *Has Not* Changed

- He denies how controlling and abusive he has been.
- He continues to blame others, including you, for his behavior.
- He demands another chance—as if it is his right and not your decision.
- He claims that you are the one who has done him wrong.
- He tries to get sympathy from you, your children, and other family and friends.
- He pressures you to move back in, attend couple counseling, or take other steps toward continuing the relationship, regardless of your own desires.
- He refuses treatment for battering, mental health, or substance abuse issues. Or you have to keep pushing him to continue with these treatments.

- He says he cannot change without your presence and support.
- He threatens suicide, violence, taking the kids, or other drastic actions.

The proof of change is whether your ex-partner can "walk the walk" and not just "talk the talk." It is much easier to talk about changing than it is to become a different person. The list above serves as a caution; those are red flags of a continuing problem with abusive control.

Signs That a Controlling or Abusive Person *Has* Changed

These changes need to last over an extended period of time to be meaningful.

- He is willing to wait however long it takes for you to trust him again. He does not pressure you to make decisions or take action until you are ready.
- He does not threaten or frighten you.
- He listens to you respectfully, even if he disagrees.
- If you say "no" to physical contact or visits, he respects your decision.
- You are free to express your opinions, anger, or frustration without being punished or shouted at in response.
- He does not try to prevent you from spending time with friends or family and does not try to punish you for your contact with others.
- He takes responsibility for his actions and does not blame you or anyone else for them.
- He admits that he behaved poorly and recognizes that this was a willful choice on his part, not a loss of control due to a "bad temper" or the influence of alcohol.
- He wants to make amends to those he has hurt for the harm he has caused.
- He is willing to continue in a battering group or other forms of counseling as long as necessary.
- Consistently, he is respectful, kind, and attentive to you (and your children) instead of acting demanding and controlling.
- He recognizes that he is responsible for his own moods and does not take out his anger and frustration on others.

- He admits to his mistakes and takes responsibility for changing his abusive behavior.

- He recognizes the controlling ways he has behaved in the past and is able to describe the effects of this control and abuse on others.

- He identifies the ways he justified his behavior in the past, and sees that these were wrong.

- He can describe his previous attitudes of entitlement and has replaced these with more empathetic and supportive views.

- He is committed to avoiding his past behavior and understands this will be a lifelong process.

- He is able to hear feedback and criticism without exploding in anger.

- If you have decided to end the relationship, he accepts the decision, even if it makes him sad. He demonstrates that he knows he cannot be in a relationship with someone who does not want to be with him, and he honors your right to make the decision.

- Regardless of his political position on gun owners' rights, if a man is serious about wanting to help his partner feel safe after a history of making her feel unsafe, he will give up his guns.

WHEN A CONTROLLING MAN
STOPS BEING PHYSICALLY VIOLENT

When a man decides to change, or attends psychotherapy or a group for batterers, he may stop his physical battering rather quickly, at least for a while. He may look like a success story—a person who is no longer violent. However, he might still try to control you in a variety of nonphysical ways. His tactics have changed, but not his dominating attitude.

When her youngest child turned 18, Bernice packed a suitcase and moved in with her parents, four hours away. Her husband, Jeff, begged her to come home. After several weeks, Bernice agreed to move back on the condition that Jeff see a psycho-therapist, attend church every Sunday, and stop hitting, pushing, or grabbing her. Jeff agreed and began therapy sessions. Bernice *told him that if he ever raised a hand to her again, she would leave him permanently. When she returned home, Jeff seemed more loving at first, but this soon faded. Despite Jeff's attending 10 psychotherapy sessions and accompanying her to church, the basic dynamic of their relationship had not changed. Jeff continued to speak harshly to Bernice, make all the decisions, and demand that Bernice build her life around his needs. Jeff never hit Bernice again, but she still did not feel safe or free.*

Even if an abusive man succeeds in stopping his physical violence, he may fail to alter his controlling attitudes and habits. Controlling mindsets are hard to change.

If your partner has gone through a change process and you feel safe enough, discuss this book with him. If you do not feel safe to do this, take this as an indicator that he still makes you feel threatened. If you continue to feel that he is testing and punishing you,

Controlling mindsets are hard to change.

then he has not changed. If he "mistakenly" tries to control you or threatens you, then he has not changed. Do not expect him to change easily. *Coercive control is a deeply rooted pattern, and it gives the controlling person certain advantages. Your partner probably will not give these up easily, and most controlling men will not give them up at all.*

9

Ending the Relationship

Deciding to end a relationship is a huge step, and a victim who makes this decision may feel frightened and alone. This chapter is addressed to people who have decided to end the coercive control relationship in which they are being victimized. It offers information about how to keep yourself safe and make sure you have help. This chapter also tells you about some of the reactions you can expect from your partner, yourself, your children, and other people when you end a controlling relationship.

A coercive control relationship is usually highly intense. Almost every moment of your day may be claimed by your abuser.

> A coercive control relationship is usually highly intense. Your abuser may claim almost every moment of your day.

Some women have found a short separation to be an important first step on their road to making a final break.

Renée, 45, was a professor of English, married to Don, 55, the head of the English department. Outwardly, they led a charmed life. They had a comfortable home, a boy and a girl, ages 10 and 11, and careers that allowed them a great deal of flexibility. They enjoyed lively conversations at the dinner table.

However, on several occasions before their children were born, Don flew into a rage and slapped Renée across the face. She once chose to cancel her classes for an entire week so she could keep the bruises secret. Since the birth of their children, Don never hit her in a way that left bruises, but he did hurt her in other ways. He was often rough with her during sex. He liked the house kept very clean, and he'd pull her by the arm to a part of the house that he thought was "a mess" and ask her to explain what had happened. He kept himself on a strict diet with no sugar, no white flour, and no meat, and insisted that Renée and the children eat the same way.

A few years into their relationship, Don announced that he wanted to feel free to have girlfriends on the side. He told Renée she should simply "overcome" her jealousy. Having grown up herself in a home where her parents fought all the time and eventually divorced, Renée was determined to keep the family intact and harmonious for her children. She was afraid to speak to people outside the family, because her husband had a prestigious position and she wanted to protect his reputation. Renée decided that she and Don would probably grow old together, and she hoped he might mellow as he aged.

One summer, Renée's sister who lived in another state asked her to visit. Renée agreed to go. The children were already scheduled to attend camp during that time, and no matter how much Don protested, Renée refused to change her mind.

A week with her sister and away from Don transformed Renée's perspective entirely. For the first couple of days she answered Don's almost constant phone calls and texts, but toward the end of the week she decided that talking once a day was plenty, and told him so. She felt freer than she had in years. The headaches and lower back pain that had plagued her disappeared. Suddenly she could imagine herself and the children living apart from Don.

After returning from her trip, Renée talked to Don about getting a divorce, and he agreed, without a lot of drama.

Other victims have described how even a short time away from their abuser has helped them see that another way of living is possible. If you can, try to take some time away from your abuser, even if it's just a few hours or one day at first. Try to resist the temptation to remain in constant contact during this time away. Time apart will help you find and listen to your own thoughts.

SEEK SUPPORT

Figure out which friends and relatives will support you and begin to tell them the truth about your relationship. Let them know what help you need. Of course not all friends and family will respond positively (see "How Others May Respond . . .," pages 176–177). The support of one or two family members or friends might give you the strength you need to live your life on your own terms.

Clara called her sister, Myrna, one day and asked if she could go to Myrna's house to discuss something urgent. Clara told Myrna about all the ways her husband, Jordan, controlled and limited her life. She had never told anyone before. The two sisters held each other and wept. Together they decided on a path to help Clara get free. They decided they would not inform their parents or other siblings until Clara had actually moved out because they could not predict how the family might react.

Myrna accompanied her sister to her first session with an advocate from the local women's center. With the advocate's help, Clara created a safety plan.

Clara set up her own bank account and had an order of protection drafted in case she needed to request it at a later point. With the support of her sister and the advocate, Clara lined up access to a nearby apartment so her children could stay in the same school district. Clara gave her sister copies of all her important documents, including her safety plan. Clara took advantage of a weekend when her husband was away, fishing with friends, to move out with her children. Her children were shocked, but she sensed that, in some way, they were also relieved.

The same weekend, after she was in the new apartment with all her boxes and her children, Clara and her sister called their mother and siblings to the new apartment and asked for their support. Seeing that her mind was made up, her family supported her. Two of Clara's brothers accompanied her to her house so she would not be alone when her husband returned from his weekend away. The three of them together told the husband about the new circumstances and told him he'd better "keep it together" for the sake of the children. And he did. He was upset and angry, but he understood that behaving well would make it easier for him to spend time with the children. He eventually entered a program for battering men, although he had never been physically violent with Clara. This program helped him understand the ways he had abusively controlled Clara. They never moved back in together. But they were able to stay friendly enough to co-parent the children from their respective homes.

Domestic Violence Agencies*

Agencies that support women in violent relationships should be helpful to you even if your partner is not physically violent. Explain the ways he controls you. Describe your concerns and fears. These agencies typically have libraries of reading materials and maybe even videos that can be helpful to you. Some also offer legal advice. And they can connect you to resources in the community. If you wish, they will assign you a counselor/advocate who will help you figure out the best path for you to take, according

> If you are in a controlling relationship with or without physical violence, domestic violence agencies should be able to help.

to your own wishes. (See the section on safety planning, pages 167–169.) Safety plans can be designed to support all types of decisions and can be changed as your decisions change.

Domestic violence agencies usually hold support group sessions for controlled and abused women. These can be tremendously empowering. Every woman's situation is different, but you are apt to find much in common as well. As you talk with the

---

*Go to *www.thehotline.org* or call 800-799-7233 (the National Domestic Violence Hotline) for advice including information about resources in your area.

other women, you will gain insight into your own situation. (See the section on police and advocates, pages 163–165.)

Therapy or Counseling

Victimized women often benefit from meeting alone with a counselor or therapist, either at the women's agency or in the community. The right therapist or counselor can help you regardless of your decision to stay or leave the relationship. Be sure to find a professional who understands coercive control. Many therapists have not yet heard of this concept and may have their own incorrect ideas about women, men, and relationships. Take this book to a session and ask the therapist to read it. Make sure the therapist truly listens to you, believes you, and helps you feel unashamed as you discuss your relationship. The right therapist can do a great deal to help you recover your self-esteem.

On the other hand, the wrong therapist might suggest that the problems in your relationship are your own fault, that you are not trying hard enough, or that you enjoy being mistreated. The wrong therapist might ignore or explain away the power imbalance. If the therapist has a bias toward preserving marriages at all costs—as do many religious counselors—the therapist might underestimate the harm of your current situation. If the therapist isn't working for you, move on. Find someone else.

Leah planned to see a psychotherapist once a week for 10 weeks, which was all her insurance covered. She found a therapist through her insurance plan. The therapist was generally supportive, and Leah began to regain some confidence. At the fourth session, Leah finally worked up enough trust to tell her therapist about Darron's constant demands and how she felt watched by him at all times. The therapist did not seem to understand the situation and offered no practical solutions. Leah felt terrible. Leah's local battered women's center recommended another therapist to her. The new therapist immediately grasped what Leah was facing and offered her the support and resources she needed to break free and recover from the controlling relationship.

Traditional couple therapy and mediation techniques do not work in relationships that involve physical violence or coercive control. They might even be dangerous. For couple therapy or mediation to be successful, each person should be able to speak freely and without fear. In situations of coercive control, one member of the couple is not entirely free. That person—usually the woman—needs her own individual support, her own therapist and/or attorney. Controlling men are often able to manipulate couple therapists and mediators into believing the woman is to blame for the problems, portraying her as unstable, paranoid, overly emotional, or even controlling. If you are caught in a controlling relationship and you agree to couple therapy or mediation, you might be placing yourself at risk.

Medical Help

Depending on your situation, a visit to a medical provider may help you out. Try to be clear about what you are seeking before you go and then tell your provider. For example:

- Do you have an injury related to your relationship?
- Do you want the person to document a bruise or other injury for a possible legal action?
- Do you want to be checked for a sexually transmitted infection or another condition?
- Do you think you might be pregnant?
- Do you have concerns about your emotional well-being, and if so, are you hoping for medication, reassurance, or a referral for counseling?
- Do you have sexual concerns related to your relationship?
- Do you need safe shelter for you and your children?
- Are you feeling physically ill from all the stress and need to address a specific symptom?

Although they should, medical providers sometimes fail to ask about situations of violence and control at home. If you want this kind of help, you'll need to let your medical provider know what's going on. Often people who are being victimized complain to their medical providers about symptoms that stem from abuse or coercive control without revealing the cause.

During several annual checkups, Elena spoke with her doctor about having trouble sleeping, gaining unwanted weight, losing interest in sex, depression, and headaches. However, she did not tell her doctor that her live-in boyfriend was pressuring her to lose weight, spat in her face during an argument, called her names, kept her away from her parents, and insisted on having intercourse with her far more often than she wanted. Her doctor suggested various treatments for each one of her symptoms but—without information about her relationship—these treatments did not help Elena find relief. Her issues were social—not medical.

Elena's situation is quite common. Many physical symptoms like the ones she reported and others, such as digestive problems and back or neck pain, are often caused by stress. A controlling or abusive relationship may be the cause of your distress. The best help will come from understanding this connection between your social situation and your body. Tell your medical provider about the source of the stress your body is expressing. Telling your medical provider what is really going on can also sometimes help you avoid expensive, unnecessary, and even harmful tests, medications, and procedures.

Unfortunately, many medical providers do not understand the needs of people in abusive and controlling relationships. For this reason, if your medical provider (or anyone else!) gives you advice, make sure the advice feels safe *to you.*

Even if you are married, your medical provider should not speak to your partner without your permission. However, if you have concerns about this, consider seeking a new provider who does not know your partner and explicitly write on your paperwork that they do not have permission to share your medical information with anyone. If you are on your partner's health insurance, he may find out about the medical consultation. He cannot find out what you and your provider discussed without your permission, but he may see a bill with the date of your visit and the name of the provider.

If you ask, your medical provider should be able to refer you to other resources in your area, such as domestic violence agencies, that can offer you other kinds of help. Remember, in every state in the United States, medical providers are mandatory reporters of child abuse (not of violence against women), and most states also require physicians to report elder abuse. If you tell a medical provider about child or elder abuse, that provider will be required to inform authorities.

Police and Advocates

If you are leaving a controlling relationship, well-trained police can assist you greatly. The officer can help you assess your safety, connect you to resources, and help you figure out what legal avenues are open to you. Their ability to act depends on the information you give them, whether crimes have been committed, and if there is evidence for these crimes.

If you decide to go to the police, you do not have to go alone. A domestic violence advocate is apt to be extremely helpful to you in getting the best possible police response. At the very least, take a friend with you as a witness. However, do not take someone who is apt to get too emotional or angry or try to speak for you.

Know the laws in your state. Some states have mandatory arrest laws and officers *must* make an arrest if they find probable cause that a domestic violence crime has occurred. If they see signs of violence, they will make an arrest even if you just want them to document the call. An advocate (or a relevant website) can let you know what your options are in your state. It is also a good idea to find out what is likely to happen and what your options are after you make a complaint. Will the abuser be arrested immediately? Can the police issue a temporary protective order until the suspect is arraigned (officially charged) in court?

What you say to the police (your statement) counts as evidence—it is important. If the police officer gives you a copy of your statement to sign, make sure you read it first. If there are any errors, make sure you correct them before you sign it. Sometimes an officer who takes a statement wants to stick to the minimal facts of a particular event. Be sure to tell the officer about previous incidents, threats, and other factors that might explain your fear and response. Also, let the officer know how your partner or ex-partner's actions made you feel. If you felt like you might die because you couldn't breathe, for instance, say it, even if the officer doesn't ask. If you feared he was going to hurt your children, because he threatened this, say so. If you give them the information, the police can document evidence of violence and threats, such as bruises, broken furniture, threatening phone messages, or signs of a break-in.

If you call the police, they are required to investigate your complaint. If you are undocumented, the police should still be able to help you without jeopardizing your immigration status. (As mentioned in Chapter 2, special visas are available to women who are victims of domestic violence.) If you choose to report to the police and are concerned about your immigration status complicating their response, ask a domestic violence advocate to accompany you.

> **If you call the police, they are required to investigate your complaint.**

If you are calling after rather than during a violent incident, you might want to call the domestic violence agency first, rather than the police, to discuss options and safety planning. You might choose not to pursue this incident through the police, at least not immediately. A safe house or a restraining order might better suit your needs.

Unfortunately, not all officers are equipped to handle situations of control and violence in intimate relationships. Some might treat you as a questionable source of evidence, rather than as a victim and a human being who has suffered. Some are insensitive and may dismiss your concerns. Seek out the police officer who is assigned to cases of domestic violence. If the department does not have a designated domestic violence officer, you may need to contact a supervisor or take an advocate with you to get the best possible response.

Advocates are often available to work in situations of sexual and domestic violence. Some are based in police departments or the prosecutor' office, while others are employed by domestic violence agencies. If you speak with an advocate, know who she is employed by and what rules she has to follow about sharing information. Usually, advocates in domestic violence agencies will communicate to the police *only* what you want, but those who work for the police or prosecutor's office directly may not be able to protect your confidentiality.

Advocates from domestic violence agencies work closely with victims and the police. They are well versed in the laws as well as local procedures. They can help you consider the advantages and disadvantages of pressing charges and what might be the best timing. They should respect your decisions about how to proceed and can help you connect with those police officers who are apt to be most compassionate and helpful.

Advocates also help victims figure out the best way to present themselves to the police, prosecutors, and the courts, so they are likely to get the outcome they want if they decide to go forward with charges.

Some women do not feel comfortable contacting the police, because their abuser is a member of the force or they have had previous negative experiences with the police. If this is your situation, contact a domestic violence agency and explore your options. If your abuser is a member of the same police department as where you are making the report, the person investigating the case should be of a higher rank than "the suspect."

HOW WILL THE ABUSER RESPOND IF YOU END THE RELATIONSHIP?

You may wonder how your partner will respond if you end the relationship. You know him—how does he tend to respond?

Proceed with caution if he's been jealous, violent, or threatening. If he has stalked you during the relationship, this is likely to continue and may get worse for a time (see "If He Stalks You," pages 173–176). If he issues a direct or veiled threat about your safety or the safety of another person, contact the police and a domestic violence advocate. Trust your instincts about the dangers to yourself and your family. You know him better than anyone else.

Prepare yourself for the ways your partner may try to prevent you from breaking off the relationship. If he has persuaded you to change your mind in the past, he is apt to use the same strategies again. And he may think up new ones. If he has tried to limit your freedom while you were together, he may not stop just because you have decided your relationship is over.

He is more likely to stop being controlling after the breakup if he feels he has a lot to lose by continuing to abuse you. If he finds a new partner, for instance, he may decide to leave you alone. However, some abusers continue to harass former partners even after the men have remarried or moved in with someone new. Some men expertly enlist their new partners in harassing their former partners, telling lies to make the new partner think the harassment is justified. If he is threatened with legal action and wants to preserve his reputation, he may leave you alone. He may not.

Patricia describes persuading Miguel to move out as "an extremely long and difficult process," with many false starts. He threatened suicide. He had a panic attack. He was drinking so much and spent so much time stalking her that he lost his job. His heart trouble worsened. He despaired. He begged to stay another year, another month, another week, another hour. Although he had not been physically violent with her in obvious ways, Patricia reached out to a counselor at the local domestic violence agency, who helped her understand that she was not responsible for fixing Miguel's problems.

Miguel remained unemployed for two years, in which he continued to send her pleading, angry, and sometimes obscene messages, even after he moved in with another woman. Finally, when he got a new job working for the town, he cared enough about his reputation to leave her alone.

Sometimes an abuser acts romantically to try to "win back" his former partner. He may give her flowers, chocolates, and cards. He may leave her adoring notes and messages. Often these romantic gestures alternate with threats and cruel statements. Try to resist these romantic strategies. Resist his attempts to "be your friend" or the desire that you might have to "be his friend." Chances are you still care about him. But a person who has been cruelly controlling with you is not apt to be content with being your friend. Maintaining any kind of contact with him will get you entangled again.

If you are worried that he might hurt himself, let other people know, but do not take this on as your responsibility. If he has access to guns, let the police know about his threats and tell them where the guns are stored.

CREATE A SAFETY PLAN

Whether you decide to stay in the relationship or leave it, a safety plan will help you. Domestic violence advocates can help you develop a plan that fits your goals and situation. Such information is also available on the Internet under the words "personalized safety plan."† If you are afraid of your partner, you will not want to tell him to leave, or tell him you are leaving, while you are alone with him. Be sure there's someone nearby who could protect you. Communicating your decision to him is just the first step. You need to know how to protect yourself, and possibly your family, into the near and distant future. Whether or not you fear physical danger, developing a careful plan will help you avoid feeling entirely alone when the relationship ends.

---

†*www.domesticviolence.org/personalized-safety-plan.*

If you need to have difficult conversations with your partner, try to hold these in a public setting such as a park or coffee shop. Avoid tough conversations in parts of the house where guns are stored or where other weapons such as knives or garden tools are easy to grab. Bathrooms, kitchens, and garages are usually dangerous places, as are bedrooms if weapons are stored there. Living rooms are apt to be safer, especially if you can stay close to a door that leads to the outside.

If you are planning to leave quickly without his awareness and are concerned about your safety, think about whether his abuse tends to follow a pattern. If so, can you plan around this pattern? If you are leaving, you'll want to leave when you know for sure that he is not around. Try to take your most important possessions with you and try to have people with you.

Almost any item could be used to physically hurt another person, including ordinary household objects such as belts and electric cords. While you cannot clear your house of these, if you have reason to fear particular items—because you have been threatened with them in the past, for instance—try to make them harder to reach. And inform the police ahead of time about the particular risks in your situation.

If Your Partner Has Access to Guns

If your partner has access to guns, you are at increased risk, even if he has never used them against you. Federal law and state statutes in the United States severely restrict and often prohibit people who are subjects of orders of protection from possessing a gun. Sometimes this even applies to situations where a *temporary* restraining order has been issued. Federal laws and state statutes usually prohibit people with domestic violence convictions (either felony or misdemeanor) from possessing a gun. These prohibitions apply even to people who would use their guns for work, such as in law enforcement, the military, corrections, or security. Of course, even with these laws on the books, many people convicted of domestic violence are still able to purchase or keep guns.

Ask your local domestic violence agency for help getting the protection you need. These laws sometimes but not always apply to long guns such as rifles used to hunt.

If your partner has guns, the following tips can help you stay safe:

- If you can, **persuade your partner to keep weapons such as guns and knives locked up** and as difficult to access as possible. Encourage your partner to keep ammunition locked up in a location separate from the guns. This reduces the likelihood of children causing an accident or of a crime committed in a sudden fit of anger. Locking up weapons keeps everyone safer.

- **Know the weapons** kept in your home, regardless of whether they are registered.

- **Keep a list** of the weapons, where they are stored, and who has access to the key, if they are locked up. Keep a copy of this list stored safely outside your home, in case you need to tell the police quickly at some point.

- If you call the police, **inform dispatch that there are guns in the home** so the responding officers can protect you and anyone else who may be present, as well as themselves.

- You may decide to **hide the guns or ammunition**, if doing so helps you make a safe getaway.

- If police have taken away the guns, **request that you be notified** when they receive a request for the return of the weapons.

- **Do not seek a gun yourself.** Naturally, many people who have been victimized think they will be safer if they themselves own a gun. Unfortunately, owning a gun is more likely to put you at risk than keep you safe, as the guns are more likely to discharge by accident or be used by an aggressor against the gun owner.

PROTECT YOUR MONEY

You may fear losing financial stability if you end your relationship. The finances of a victim who separates from her abuser usually improve with time, but this initial insecurity is scary. If you think there is any possibility that your partner will try to take advantage of you financially, protect yourself. It is usually best to close joint banks accounts and open up an account in your own name. Change the passwords and PINs on all your accounts. Even if you never shared them with your abuser, he may know what they are. Close your joint credit cards if you think there is any possibility that he will try to run up charges in your name. If he has betrayed you financially, seek help from the banks and an attorney. Your local women's center can probably refer you to help in this regard.

Finances are often a problem for women who set out on their own, especially if they have children to support. You may need to apply for public assistance for a time. You may need to rely on relatives or find a new job. Things will get better.

Try to have a financial plan lined up before you leave so you will be less likely to feel forced to return for financial reasons.

Margie bought and stored at a friend's home the household items she would need when she moved out, including bedding, towels, cleaning supplies, and small appliances. She also hid her best jewelry and important documents at her friend's house, just to be safe. These steps helped Margie have the confidence to tell her boyfriend, Rod, that she was leaving. She told him in the presence of two friends who had accompanied her for this purpose. When Rod grew angry, Margie and the friends told him that he needed to calm down and understand the situation. She had scheduled a truck to pick up her belongings that afternoon. One of the friends waited with Rod so he would not do anything irrational. Margie was glad she had prepared in advance.

> **Make a financial plan before you leave so you won't be forced to return for monetary reasons.**

The exact process around leaving, telling your partner the relationship is over, and collecting your stuff or getting him to move out can be both complicated and dangerous. Some women prefer to "just get out" and worry about their possessions later. Others who have left without their belongings later regret not collecting their most valued items. Only you can know the best way for you to leave or to ask him to leave. A domestic violence advocate will offer you support. Advocates have a lot of experience in this area, know the relevant laws, and can help you get police protection if you need it.

PROTECT YOUR CHILDREN

Many women fear that their children's lives will become much worse if they end a relationship of coercive control. Sometimes this is true for the short term. In the long term the children are happier if their mother is happier. Women typically become better mothers when they are free to consider their own needs and are not afraid for their safety. Also, when children see one member of a couple controlling the other, they grow up thinking that this is how people should relate to each other. They are apt to carry these patterns into their own relationships. A man who exerts coercive control with his partner is often inappropriately controlling with the children, too. For all these reasons and more, women should think twice before deciding to stay in a controlling relationship "for the children."

Children need help with big transitions. Children often become angry at their mothers when their mothers end their relationships, especially if the controlling man is the children's father or father figure. Because the mother feels like a safer parent, the children will often turn their feelings of rage toward her while continuing to try to please the father. Naturally, this is upsetting to mothers who are working so hard to keep their children safe.

Allow your children to express their feelings—whether these are anger, sadness, confusion, or something else. At the same time, if they are calling you names or in other ways mistreating you, feel free to tell them that this is not acceptable. *It is better for your children, as well as you, for them not to abuse you.* Find a therapist who is knowledgeable about children, separation, and divorce. Comfort your children if they are sad. If they are angry, they probably also need your comfort, but may not be sure how to ask for it or be willing to accept it openly. Some mothers are able to comfort even angry children by leaving them simple loving notes, showing them affection, and checking in with them frequently about their activities and feelings.

Many children benefit from speaking with other young people whose parents have recently divorced or separated. Some schools or community centers have such support groups. If your children are in a school with a guidance counselor, psychologist, or social worker, see if they are running such a group or would be willing to start one. Even just a few group sessions can be tremendously liberating for children. Many women's centers run discussion groups for children.

> **Children benefit from meeting with others whose parents have recently divorced or separated.**

Probably, you will also benefit from speaking with a variety of mothers who have been in a similar situation. Trust your own judgment if they offer you advice. What works for one woman or family may not work for another.

If your partner or ex-partner has been violent with the children, or if you fear for their physical safety, you may want to seek assistance from neighbors, your children's school, and family members. Let them know your concerns. Ask them to report anything unusual to the police. If safe and appropriate, ask them to speak to your partner or ex-partner. If you tell someone about your partner abusing a child, that person may call child protective services. This could work for or against you.

Some women contact child protective services themselves and report that their partner has put the children at risk. This could be tricky—many women have been blamed by child protective services for failing to protect their children from a violent man. Generally, child protective service workers are more knowledgeable these days than they used to be about the needs of women who are subject to violence and control.

If you and your partner share small children, ending a violent or controlling relationship raises concerns about custody and visitation. Your local domestic violence agency can help you with this. Here are some options:

- If you have sole custody of your children but a judge has ordered some type of visitation, you can ask for **special conditions**, such as supervised visits only, or a requirement that their father cannot drink or use drugs when with the children, or that certain dangerous people cannot be with him when the children are visiting.
- **Choose a neutral pickup site** or have others drop off and pick up your children. This may help you keep where you live secret.
- If you have a protective order or you don't think it is safe to be in the same place alone with their father, consider choosing a **public place to meet for visitation exchanges**. A police station, restaurant, or other public setting is a good choice.
- In extreme cases you can ask the court to appoint a **visitation supervision monitor**. They will arrange for the drop-off and pickup to be staggered in time, with the monitor watching the children in between. Some domestic violence agencies have visitation centers where either the exchange of children or the entire visit can be supervised.
- If you have other ideas about how visitation can be handled to minimize hassle and risk for yourself and the children, suggest your plan to the judge.

IF HE STALKS YOU

Many men continue to engage in controlling and intimidating behaviors even after their wife or girlfriend makes it clear the relationship is over. If these efforts for contact are one-sided, this is called "persistent pursuit," which is a form of stalking. Persistent pursuit can be unsettling or even terrifying. It usually lessens over time and lasts about two years[7] on average. Stalking is a crime, and police are growing increasingly skilled at pursuing it. Most stalkers are male former intimate partners of the person they are stalking. And most stalking victims are women.[8]

Usually, men who stalk do so in multiple ways. Knowing his ex-partner well, the stalker knows how to hurt her. He will reach the woman where he can: through her family, children, friends, home, workplace, or through the courts. He might initiate contact, spread rumors, follow her, send her indecent messages or objects, break into her home, move into her neighborhood, hack her computer, call her multiple times a day, and so on. Many of these behaviors are considered criminal harassment or other crimes.

After he moved out, Nate stalked Elizabeth for more than two years. He sprinkled flower petals on her driveway, extended the process of picking up his possessions, sent numerous harassing e-mails, tracked her movements, involved her in a court case, spread rumors around town, and came onto her property when she'd asked him not to. He broke into her office and propped up a picture of himself on her desk. He began dating and quickly moved in with the only single woman in her office, using his connection with his new girlfriend to continue stalking her.

Looking back, Elizabeth wished she had had the strength to tell Nate to leave earlier and had cut off all contact completely on the day he moved out. At the time of their breakup, Elizabeth still loved Nate and was trying to "be nice." She had been raised to be nice, and she thought that by pleasing Nate she might help him act more reasonably. She was also afraid of Nate's anger. Elizabeth eventually followed the counselor's advice to ignore all Nate's efforts to contact her. As the months passed, he contacted her less and less often and, eventually, he left her alone.

Three years after his departure, Elizabeth found a webcam hidden in the bedroom clock. It had been installed by Nate years earlier. The police determined that it no longer contained the chip for recording. Nate's behaviors definitely constituted a variety of crimes including stalking and criminal harassment. Working with the detective who specialized in domestic violence, Elizabeth developed a plan for pressing charges if Nate ever contacted her again.

A man who stalks a woman after a breakup often begins stalking her while they are still together: following her from room to room and outside, hacking her computer, and making her account for her whereabouts. Fortunately, the legal system is increasingly recognizing these behaviors that occur within a relationship as stalking.

A controlling man who feels rejected may try to sabotage his ex-partner's ability to have romantic relationships.

Hank knew that his former wife, Cindy, had joined a dating service. He set up several accounts on the service, using names, photographs, and descriptions that he figured she would find attractive. He then corresponded with her from these various accounts, posing as other men. He tried to make her feel bad by arranging dates and not showing up, and by sending sexually inappropriate messages. Since Hank had also hacked Cindy's account, he was able to send off-putting messages to the real potential suitors Cindy encountered, making her despair about the dating pool. She resigned from the dating service. A few months later, Hank moved in with a new girlfriend and became heavily involved with her and her family. He left Cindy alone. Eventually, Cindy met a new man whom she grew to trust over time.

Stalking is a crime. However, it can be difficult to prosecute successfully. Many abusers use a range of secret tactics, such as installing spyware on a computer or setting up hidden cameras. Other actions look unremarkable to others, but the abused person knows they are intended as a message or a threat. *If you are stalked, be sure to record every incident with as much information as possible, including the dates, times, potential witnesses, and exactly what happened. Also record what you did in response, and any contacts you may have with the police.* If there are any witnesses, be sure to note this, too. Even if you do not want to pursue legal charges at this point, keeping a record will help you later, if you change your mind or if the situation worsens.

Stalking can be so terrifying and confusing that many victims will agree to meet with their former partner, to see if they can be friends or try to persuade him to leave them alone. Some

victims even have sex with their stalkers, or resume the relationship, figuring that this might be a way to calm him down and get
on his good side—keeping them safer. Unfortunately, engaging
with a stalker may weaken any later efforts to gain police protection. Stalkers know this—it is part of their strategy.

HOW OTHERS MAY RESPOND IF YOU END
THE RELATIONSHIP

Your friends, family, coworkers, and neighbors may not understand what has happened when you separate from the person who
has been controlling you. For years you may have been putting up
a front, pretending everything was okay, and looking happy with
this person. The abuser is unlikely to have revealed his controlling side in public. In what may look like an overnight switch,
suddenly you are talking to others about feeling afraid of your
ex-partner and feeling controlled by him. Others may hesitate to
accept the reality of the coercive control in the relationship. They
may continue being friends with your abuser. Some people may
choose to side with your abuser rather than you. You may lose
some friends—at least temporarily—over the breakup. His relatives (and maybe even some of your relatives) may stop speaking
with you. All this hurts. Over time it will hurt less, and some of
these people may return to you.

Ida's mother always liked Ida's second husband, Damien, and was
disappointed when Ida told her she was getting divorced. Damien
was 15 years older than Ida, and acted charming in public. Ida's
mother had thought Damien would take care of Ida and the
children from her first marriage. Ida's mother listened to Ida's
stories about the control and abuse she was subjected to, seemed
to understand them, and expressed her sympathy. And yet, she
could not seem to accept how bad things had been. "He was just
jealous because you are so young and pretty," she'd say when Ida
described the spyware she had found on her computer. "Just tell

him he's frightening you," she advised her daughter when Ida told her about the strange e-mails he sent her. "Mom, he's trying to frighten me," Ida would reply. While most of her friends immediately grasped what had happened and sided with her, Ida felt sad that her mother could not or would not. Her mother insisted it was just a misunderstanding, and that he had stalked and threatened her simply because he loved her so much.

Because of their own issues, some people will never understand or accept the reality of your experiences. Although it's painful to be abandoned or mistreated by people who do not seem to understand, try not to let your fear of their opinions prevent you from living your authentic life. You may also be surprised by the support you receive from people who *do* understand.

Jill and Eduardo had been friends with Ida for years when she became involved with Damien, who became increasingly controlling. The two couples occasionally enjoyed dinners together and played cards. When they broke up, Damien called Jill and tried to tell her what an awful person Ida was and how all his actions were justified. Jill cut him off immediately and told Damien, "We have been friends with Ida for years and do not want to hear you say bad things about her. Don't call us again." Jill and Eduardo helped Ida get through the especially rocky two years in which Damien stalked her.

FINAL THOUGHTS ON ENDING A RELATIONSHIP OF COERCIVE CONTROL

Wherever you are in the process of leaving a controlling relationship, remember that the intensity of the feelings will fade over time. Get support. Have hope. You will be able to be free and also happy. But it will take time. Be patient with yourself. Be kind to yourself. Spend time only with people who make you feel good about yourself. You have been through a lot.

In summary, if you are being coercively controlled in a relationship, and you want to end the relationship:

1. Look carefully at the relationship with your new understanding of coercive control.
2. Get support.
3. Make a safety plan.
4. Execute your plan.
5. Keep contact to a minimum.
6. Continue to get support long after you separate.
7. Expect that it may take you a long time to fully recover.
8. Know that you will recover.

IF THE ABUSER ENDS THE RELATIONSHIP

Some controlling people take the initiative themselves to end the relationship. The moment may arrive suddenly and be unexpected, or the abuser may hint over time that the day is coming. The abuser held you tight and kept you close for a while. Now, with similar resolve, he pushes you away or cuts you off entirely. The rejection hurts.

Controlling men often end relationships selfishly and cruelly. They may leave because they have found another woman who is younger, richer, or more obedient, or in some way seen as more desirable. They may leave because they are bored. It's important to understand that these decisions are a reflection of the abuser's ego and selfishness—it is not a true comment on his partner's value.

Many controlling men will do everything they can to hurt their partners on their way out the door—for instance, blaming and insulting her, stealing her money or other possessions, raping her, or getting her pregnant against her will. Being left behind hurts a woman's self-esteem even when she knows the relationship had been problematic. Being rejected can leave a woman feeling worthless and even suicidal. The situation will look different to her in a year or two. It will take time to adjust.

Miriam's husband, Dirk, was a surgeon. They lived on a farm with hens, a couple of horses, and two dairy cows. Miriam stayed home with their four children, who were all under six years old. Her youngest was just two months old. One morning when Miriam woke up, Dirk was gone. He had left a note saying simply, "Bye." Miriam panicked. She discovered that he had drained their bank accounts and cut off their credit cards. She alone had to care for their four children and all their animals. Miriam found out that Dirk had run off with a young resident from the hospital. As painful as this was, Miriam couldn't understand why he chose to inflict additional pain not just on her but also on the children, by leaving her with no money. Although he had barely been involved in his children's lives, Dirk fought Miriam for full custody of them. When she was granted custody and Dirk was told he would have to pay child support, he fled to Canada. Miriam raised the children alone. She set up a family daycare in her home. Although the years immediately following the separation were a huge struggle, Miriam created a happy, stable home for herself and her children.

In the hours, days, and months following the departure of a controlling man, a woman might think she cannot survive on her own. During these times, it is especially important to reach out to others for help.

I wish you the strength to seek your freedom. I wish you safety. And I wish you much support on your journey.

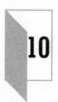

Feeling Like Yourself Again
RECOVERING FROM COERCIVE CONTROL

Just as two people come together as a couple in stages marked by important moments, relationships often dissolve in stages too. Some people's exit from a relationship is abrupt and definitive—we can think of it as turning away and never looking back. But more often the end of a relationship feels like two steps forward and one step back, until it is truly "over."

If you have been in a coercive control relationship, you will notice yourself passing through a series of phases as you recover. You may well experience periods of crisis at the beginning. Over time, these will become less frequent until you realize you have your life back and you are feeling like yourself again. Envision having your life back. Taste it if you can. Know that it can be yours. But first, you'll need to get through the rough part.

HOW YOU MAY FEEL IF YOU END THE RELATIONSHIP

You are apt to feel a jumble of emotions at the end of a relationship of coercive control. On one hand, you may feel liberated,

180

picturing yourself living in a freer way—able to make decisions on your own, speak with whomever you like, and control your own time. This glimpse of freedom may make you happy.

However, the end of any relationship brings feelings of grief and loss. Your life may seem to be a complete mess. Sorting out issues such as finances and child visitation takes time. Even the best separations can feel like a crisis for many months. And although the pain will lessen, it may not vanish entirely for years.

You may worry about the effects of the separation on your children (see "Protect Your Children," pages 171–173). Many people feel sad looking back on the time they spent with their ex-partner and wonder if it was all wasted. They think back on the happy times and wonder what to do with those memories. Should they just delete them, somehow, like digital photos from a phone or computer? But the memories—both good and bad—do leave a trace.

You may grapple with feelings of shame as you recall how you behaved or what you tolerated under your ex-partner's influence. The shame stems from the abuser's manipulations, and you will outgrow it. You may wonder why you stayed as long as you did. You may feel afraid that your ex-partner will come after you, your children, or others you love. And to make matters worse, your ex-partner might be stalking you by calling, texting, showing up at your home or workplace, or sending letters or e-mails.

You may feel afraid to break off all contact, because you think it is safer to keep him in your sights. Like many women, you may want to find a way to be "friends" with an intimate partner who has controlled you. You may still feel responsible for managing his feelings. You may think that being friendly with him will keep him from becoming angry and dangerous. Most women discover over time that being friendly with a controlling or abusive man keeps a dangerous door open, and leaves them vulnerable to getting hurt. Keeping contact to a minimum is your best strategy. If you do not share young children, try to see if you can cut off the connection altogether. This will help both of you move on.

Keep contact to a minimum after the relationship ends.

Shortly after you have ended the relationship, try to focus your thoughts on the bad parts of it. This will prevent you from falling under your ex-partner's control again. This is not the time to remember all the happy moments or to look over photos that highlight fun and loving events.

You may not know what to do with yourself without your partner's demands.

After her breakup, Alicia felt as if her days had no direction. When she had lived with George, she knew that her main goal was to make him happy. Despite the frustrations, at least she felt her life had a purpose. When she finally broke off their relationship because she could not bear to be under his control, she felt as if she was just "floating through" her days.

Like Alicia, you may have lost the feeling that you had a mission and purpose in life. The plans you set with your ex-partner no longer hold; this may leave you with a big question mark in your future. You will eventually make new plans, but it will take some time to see the road ahead of you clearly. You may suffer from nightmares or anxiety, and sleep and eat too much or too little. Don't hesitate to seek a counselor or therapist to help you through this particularly difficult period.

Remember, you have done nothing wrong in deciding to end a relationship with a controlling person. This is your right. Even if you are making your ex-partner unhappy and unsettling your children, you have the right to decide how you want to live your life. Think about yourself and your own healing.

Even after they have left a controlling relationship, many women experience strong feelings in response to events, people, or places that remind them of the controlling man. One woman found herself becoming unduly angry when her new boyfriend asked her, casually, where she had spent the afternoon. Another burst into tears when a male coworker raised his voice.

Suzy felt anxious when she was late getting home from work, even though she knew her ex-husband, Jeremy, was no longer at home to shout at her. Suzy also preserved certain rigid habits instilled by Jeremy—always keeping "his" side of the sink clear, carefully putting away her clothes before she went to bed, and worrying excessively if her house was not entirely neat. She felt these behaviors were not "hers" but rather had been imposed by Jeremy. Still, it took Suzy a couple of years to be able to tolerate the fear and discomfort that came over her when she was not conforming to Jeremy's exacting standards. Over time, she began to feel free to keep a neat house (or not) in response to her own desires, rather than the echo of Jeremy's demands.

Transitioning from a controlling relationship is a slow and bumpy process. Some women become emotional while listening to songs, watching movies, or speaking with friends. Be patient with yourself and know you will come to feel more stable again.

Forgiving?

Sometimes friends, family, and religious leaders will push you to forgive the person who has controlled and hurt you. They may describe this as a moral obligation. Their position may make you feel controlled all over again! They are telling you how you should think and feel. You've had enough of that. Gently let them know that you need to come to your own feelings at your own pace. Even if it takes longer than you would like and even if it never comes, forgiveness cannot be rushed or forced. Some things may not be forgivable, ever. You will ultimately recover

> Forgiveness cannot be rushed or forced. You may never forgive certain acts. You will recover from the abuse even if you do not forgive the abuser.

from the abuse even if you never forgive the abuser. Forgiveness usually comes after a couple of years, if it comes at all.

Controlling men seldom sincerely admit to having done wrong or humbly ask for pardon. Instead they often *demand* forgiveness. Or they act as if their "sorry" means they are no longer responsible for the hurt they caused. You have a right to lingering feelings of anger for all you have been through.

In some cases the person who has wronged you might be suffering, suicidal, or dying. People may try to persuade you that forgiving him is essential to his well-being. They want everything to be "back to normal." Please know, your abuser can engage in his own process of recovery without your forgiveness. Do not feel obligated to take care of him again in this way. Some questions to ask yourself:

- What might you gain from forgiving your abuser? Are you ready to forgive? What risks might be involved in forgiving him?
- Is he truly sorry? How do you know? What efforts has he made to communicate that he is sorry? Does this differ from other times he may have asked forgiveness, only to do the same thing again?
- Does his feeling of being sorry last over time, or does it alternate with anger and entitlement?
- Does he understand how he hurt you (and possibly others), or is he sorry only because he lost you? In other words, is he regretful because he has done wrong, or because he has lost a relationship or a lifestyle that he enjoyed?
- Has he tried to make amends for all the wrong he has done you (and possibly your children)? Of course, there is no way to "pay back" for time lost or years of suffering. However, some former abusers who truly feel sorry do try to atone for their past misdeeds by making real sacrifices to enable their children or former partner to go back to school, have therapy, or simply live more comfortably. This would be a way of making amends. Some men who had once been controlling make amends by becoming active in combating violence against women.

Even if your former partner sincerely seems to want to make amends, his being sorry does not require any action—including forgiveness—on your part. Even if he is apologetic and appears to have changed, you have no obligation toward him.

If you do decide to forgive the person who has controlled you, do not assume that this means you should be willing to enter the relationship again. Some women find it helpful to allow themselves to feel regret rather than forgiveness. They may regret that the relationship did not work out and regret that they could not have the life together that they'd once imagined. They may regret that they were deprived of their dreams by the other person's disrespectful and unkind treatment. They may also feel regret if the abuser is not doing so well after the separation, but they should not feel guilty about this. Remember, *his* behavior caused the separation.

After a couple of years, some former victims do decide to forgive their abuser because it helps them move on with their own feelings and their own lives. This forgiveness might be private, or it might be shared only with a counselor or an intimate friend. It is risky to let the controlling person know that you have forgiven him—he might see this as a window to get back into your life. Whether or not you decide to forgive, this decision should be about your well-being—not the well-being of your abuser.

SOME TIPS FOR RECOVERING FROM A COERCIVE CONTROL RELATIONSHIP

People who have been victimized come up with their own paths toward recovery. What is helpful for one person may not be helpful for another. This list is intended to suggest some possibilities to you. By all means, come up with your own!

• **Become re-involved in activities that the controlling person would not allow you to do.** For instance, Lisa's partner would not allow her to ride a bicycle. She bought a used bicycle and felt a wave of liberation every time she rode it. Cynthia's husband did not want her wearing makeup. She asked a friend to help her choose lipstick and eyeliner and gradually began wearing these again.

• **Reestablish relationships with family and friends from whom the controlling person had isolated you.** Make a list of the people with whom you have lost contact and see if you can reestablish the bonds. Be cautious, however, about contacting former romantic partners too soon.

- **Surround yourself with people who support you.** Spend time with people who make you feel good about yourself and lift you up. Try to avoid those people who bring you down.

- **Sort through your possessions.** If you have clothes, books, furniture, and other items from the controlling relationship, you may find it helpful to give these away. Many people cannot do this all at once, but with each item they replace, they feel freer and freer.

- **Counseling or psychotherapy** can help you understand the relationship that you have ended and will help you face the challenges ahead. A good psychotherapist will also help you feel less alone, and will help you improve your relationships with other people.

- **Consider becoming an activist on social issues that are important to you**. Former victims feel empowered as they make their voices heard. For instance, "take back the night" marches are held annually in many cities and towns. In these marches women and men proclaim women's right to live without violence. People who were once victims feel visible and empowered when they march in protests and engage in letter-writing campaigns and other forms of activism and community education.

- **Express yourself creatively**. Do you like to dance? Write? Draw? Garden? Sing? Cook? Find a way to express yourself. Many victims shut down creatively during the coercive control relationship. Maybe their partner criticized their work, or maybe they felt too frightened to express themselves. Maybe they were just too busy attending to their partner's demands. Leaving a controlling relationship might help release your artistic side. See if you can find an outlet.

- **Reclaim your body by becoming physically active.** Try something you've enjoyed in the past, or experiment with something new. Walking, yoga, dancing, lifting weights, bopping to the radio while you cook a meal—physical activity can help you feel your vitality again.

- **Consider a medical check-up**. Did you neglect your health during the relationship? Do you have unresolved medical issues? Should you be checked for a sexually transmitted infection or an injury? Do you want to give up an unhealthy habit? Having a medical provider say you are okay, or help you get the treatment you need to get better, is a step on your road to recovery.

- **Make a list of the controlling incidents and practices that you experienced.** You will probably not be able to remember these all at once. Keep adding to it over time. You can refer to the list when you doubt your memories or your interpretation of events. The list will also help you appreciate what you've been through and see how strong you are.

- **Be optimistic that recovery will happen** . . . even if it is not as fast as you want.

- **Read relevant materials** (see the Resources at the back of the book).

- **Be kind to yourself.** For a while after your relationship, you may hear the abuser's voice in your head, telling you that you cannot do anything right, you are stupid or ugly or whatever he would say. You need to replace that voice with a kind one. If you do something well, no matter how small, tell yourself, "Nice job!" If something does not turn out as well as you would have liked, tell yourself, "Okay, this is how I learn. No one's perfect."

- **Be patient with yourself.** Recovery may take a long time.

- **Focus more on yourself.** As often as you can, ask yourself, "How am I feeling now? What do I feel like doing now?" Of course, you may not always be able to do what you want. But just being able to identify what you feel like doing is important, after you have focused for a long while exclusively on the needs of another person. Do things that bring you pleasure and that are good for you.

- **Look ahead, not behind, as much as possible.** Take pride in the courage you showed and look forward to a full life of freedom, friends, and family.

- **Separate yourself entirely from the controlling person and anyone who interacts with him,** as much as possible, so he cannot seek to control or monitor you through someone else.

- **Share your story,** when and how it feels right to you. Telling your story can help you cope with your feelings about the experience, and may also have positive practical effects. For instance, if your boss understands the situation, your ex-partner may not be able to cause so much trouble for you at work. If you tell friends, they will understand you better and may be able to offer support. You need to assess your safety and comfort in this, making sure you speak about it only to those who are likely to support you.

ENTERING A NEW RELATIONSHIP

It takes many former victims of coercive control a long time to trust others fully again. Nevertheless, some women do rush into a new relationship when the controlling one ends because they miss the companionship and security that even an abusive relationship provided. If you head into a new relationship before you are ready, you might doom the new relationship to failure. Many women know this, but rush into a new relationship anyway, drawn to the promise of love and protection.

> It may take you a long time to trust others fully again.

When a woman who has been in a controlling relationship meets a possible new partner, it is important that she ask herself if this new partner is showing signs of being controlling, too. Here are some questions to consider:

- Do you feel obligated to spend more time with him than you would like?
- Is he asking you for a commitment before you are ready, such as dating exclusively, living together, getting married, or having a baby?
- Does he want to take over aspects of your life such as your parenting, your home, or your money?
- Does he treat you as an inferior?
- Does he seem too eager to win over your children, parents, or friends?
- Has he ever hurt you physically?
- Has he knowingly hurt you during sex?
- Does he act possessive and jealous?
- When you say "no" to something, does he try to push you?
- Does he ever make you feel afraid?
- Does he abuse alcohol and/or drugs?
- Does he seem to lack empathy for others?
- Does he lack respect for other people's opinions?
- Does he disregard the impact of his behavior on you and others?
- Does he blame his behavior on others?
- Does he speak disrespectfully about his past partners?
- In general, does he treat people poorly?
- Does he ignore your needs, your schedule, your opinions, and your life?
- Do you feel trapped? Do you feel invaded?
- Does he make you feel ashamed of yourself?

If you answered "yes" to any of the questions above, your new relationship may be headed for trouble. Maybe this is because your new partner is controlling. Or maybe you have not expressed what you want clearly, after having learned to ignore your own needs when you were with your controlling partner. Try to let your new partner know what you need and want. How he responds will help you decide whether this person is right for you.

Your new partner should respect that you may need more time and space alone than other women, because of your experiences under coercive control. If the new relationship is going to succeed, he must learn to respect your boundaries.

Your new partner might be tempted to attack the person who has wronged you. Although his feelings of anger are natural, a verbal or physical confrontation would not help you in the long run and might put you at further risk. Encourage him to focus on helping you, rather than on hurting the person who has wronged you.

If Someone You Care About Is Being Victimized by Coercive Control

It is hard to watch a friend, family member, client, or patient suffer at the hands of a controlling partner or ex-partner. You may feel like rescuing the victim. You may feel like killing the abuser. You may get so frustrated that you want to walk away. It may make you weep with anger or sadness. Long-term patterns of abuse and control usually require long-term patterns of assistance before the victim can escape.

Controlling relationships have their ups and downs. Victims will be more willing to discuss the problems openly—and think about making changes—during a phase when they can feel the tension building or immediately after there has been a particularly bad episode. On the other hand, during times when the controlling man is acting sorry and doing his best to make his wife or girlfriend feel loved and cared for, she is unlikely to be open to discussing the relationship's problems or to think about leaving.

Remember, the victim's self-esteem has likely been hurt by the abuse and the isolation. She may be at greater risk of physical danger than you realize. Her conversations, movements, and electronic communications may be monitored. You cannot "make" her break free until she is ready. To do so might put her (and possibly you) at risk. However, the following may help:

- **Let her know your concerns in a nonjudgmental way**. Over time, if you are close enough to the woman and you are sure your conversation is not being monitored, describe what makes you concerned.

- **Ask what you can do to help, but do not take over**. Ask what you can do that would make her life easier and give her strength. Do not commit to more than you can actually take on.

- **Avoid telling her what to do.** Remember, she is the expert on her situation. She can assess her safety better than anyone else.

- **Listen to what she wants to tell you and resist throwing too many questions at her.** Some parts of what she has been through may make her feel ashamed. It may take years before she is ready to share the most painful parts of her relationship.

- **Give her a copy of this book if she has a safe place to keep it.** If it feels comfortable, ask her questions about how this book applies to her life. Gently share your impressions.

- **Allow her to express a range of feelings without criticism**. She may still love her partner or ex-partner and believe he loves her. She may miss him. She may feel dependent on him and wonder how she is going to survive without him. She may be worried about his well-being. Reassure her that all these feelings are normal and they will sort themselves out over time. Even if you think this man is a jerk and there is nothing good about him, do not criticize him too harshly or she may be ashamed to tell you about the ways she still feels attached to him. She may resent you for criticizing so harshly someone she still loves. Remember, she might return to him. If she does, you want her to feel comfortable staying in touch with you.

If she seems to be completely under her partner's control, there may not be much you can do for now other than stay connected and gently help her see times when the abuser's words do not match his actions. She has most likely been through more than she has told you.

ESPECIALLY FOR FAMILY AND FRIENDS

Friends and family members have a vitally important role in helping a loved one who is in a relationship of coercive control. You are in the best position to stay connected with the victim socially and help her feel good about herself. Just by being with her, you remind her of who she is outside the relationship. You help her form and remember her own opinions and perspectives. Your connection helps her feel valued and less alone. When you treat her with respect, you help her feel like herself again. By helping her feel valuable and capable, you counteract some of the messages she receives from her abuser.

While your friendship is important, you should probably try not to give too much advice. Advocates who work with controlling and abusive relationships every day will be able to offer the best advice about safety planning. For example, many people tell their friends to obtain a restraining order. For some victims, this is highly dangerous and might lead to increased violence.

Encourage your loved one to seek professional support from a women's agency or domestic violence service provider. Bring her to her first appointment if she wants, but allow her to meet with the advocate alone. If she is anxious or depressed, she may also benefit from the help of a counselor or psychotherapist who understands controlling relationships. If she is afraid, she may need to call the police. These choices are hers to make.

If she has children, she probably worries about how she will manage with them alone if the relationship ends. If you can offer concrete help—such as housing, babysitting, or money—let her know. If the children can live with you for a time, let her know. Again, do not offer more than you can actually manage.

FOR PROFESSIONALS IN THE FIELD

You are probably working with someone who has various complaints but has not put them together under the label of "coercive control." Whether you work in law enforcement, social services, mental health, medicine, or other fields, the following questions may help you figure out when coercive control is present. Of course, these need to be asked of a potential victim in a private setting.

- Is someone controlling you?
- Is someone hurting you?
- Do you feel threatened?
- Are you afraid to speak up?
- How can I help?
- What do you need?

People in mental health, social work, and medicine might want to ask additional questions such as:

- Do you feel alone and isolated?
- Is someone tracking where you go and what you do?
- Do you feel like a free person? If not, why not?
- Is someone manipulating you?
- Does someone make you feel badly about yourself?
- Are you in a relationship that is hurting your health or well-being?

Sometimes it is difficult for professionals to understand the psychological control an abuser wields over his victim. Police and other first responders often grow frustrated with domestic violence calls. The abuser poses a real threat, but he may appear to outsiders to be calmer than the victim, because he is not afraid.

Although others may not understand her logic, an abused woman is often the best expert at weighing and minimizing the risks to herself and her children. She might maintain or resume contact with the abuser in an attempt to soothe his feelings and reduce his threatening behavior.

Tova was being stalked by Tony, who had been extremely controlling and somewhat violent in their years together. Tova ignored his phone calls, letters, e-mails, and texts. One day, Tova's parents called her and told her that Tony had appeared at their house, threatening to "blow the place up" unless they talked some sense into their daughter and made her "come home." Tova called Tony immediately to tell him to leave her parents out of it. He had found the key to getting her to respond by threatening her parents, and he began to involve others in his harassment of Tova.

The victim—who is both controlled by the abuser and terrified—may fail to cooperate with investigations or prosecutions. She may continue living with the abuser, seeing this as the safest route for herself and her children. She may seem to pardon much of what he does because he calls it "love."

We have to be careful not to blame the person who is being victimized. Sometimes professionals misread the situation right in front of their eyes. They see a woman who has broken away and is being stalked by her abuser—and still they blame the victim for not getting away.

The social and criminal justice systems often fail the abused women they are supposed to protect. After a violent episode, too many assaultive men are arrested and promptly released. They return home angrier than ever. Victims who try to file reports may be made to wait for hours, or asked what they had done to provoke the incidents, or told they "have no case" because there is no documented physical abuse or no physical evidence of stalking. A mother who seeks assistance may suddenly find herself answering social workers' questions about her "failure to protect" her child. She feels blamed, while no one confronts the abuser.

Police, judges, therapists, and child custody evaluators are often fooled by the controlling man, who seems calm and reasonable compared to the victimized woman. She has been frustrated, frightened, and agitated by the abuse. He actively develops an image as a "nice guy with a crazy woman." Therapists, medical personnel, and social workers may fall for his tricks and label the woman as hysterical, masochistic, overly emotional, or even controlling.

> A controlling person maintains calm while his frightened ex-partner looks "overly emotional."

If professionals in the field fail to ask the right questions about the controlling dynamics, they will not be able to offer meaningful help. Often, in fact, professionals unwittingly side with the controlling man, deepening the woman's isolation.

Domestic violence advocates usually do understand the dynamics of controlling relationships, since they have daily contact with people victimized by coercive control as well as physical violence. Advocates enable women to expand their freedom within the relationship, or find safe routes of escape, if necessary.

Professionals often think they know what's best. It can be difficult to resist the temptation to tell a person who is being abused and controlled what to do. To the outside, it may appear simple: she should leave the relationship, file charges, cut off all contact, and so forth. However noble our intentions, telling a person who is suffering from control what to do is perpetrating another form of control against her. She understands the complexities and risks better than anyone else. We must stop ourselves from crossing the line that separates "helping" from "taking over." The best approach is to ask respectful questions, provide resources and options, and allow the victimized person to make her own decisions at all times. If you respect her choices and judgment, you will help her recover her confidence and her ability to direct her own life.

We must understand how terrifying stalking is. Many stalking behaviors can be interpreted in more than one way, and may look "innocent" to an outsider, but the victim understands their true intent. For instance, if a stalker leaves a rose and a love note on the car of his ex-wife, this may look to some like a romantic gesture. However, the stalker has demonstrated that he knows where she is and is unafraid to touch her property. He has also demonstrated that he does not accept her ending the relationship.

We should take victims' accounts of stalking seriously, even if they seem unbelievable or unlikely. She hears noises in the night, objects appear and disappear in her home or yard, her computer acts strange, items are delivered to her house that she did not order, friends stop speaking with her, her stalker appears on the street and in other public places but then vanishes, and so on. A woman often hesitates to tell these stories to others because she believes

> **Stalking terrifies victims, in part because it is so unpredictable.**

they make her sound crazy. We must remember that some abusers go to great lengths to make their victim seem crazy. That is their strategy.

New technologies that can be used for stalking emerge all the time. What seems impossible one day is routine and affordable the next. Ordinary-appearing digital clocks hold small cameras, computer webcams can be activated from a distance, listening and tracking devices are easily installed in cell phones, and numerous programs track a victim's computer activity. We cannot even imagine what will be available tomorrow. If a victim talks about being tracked or spied upon by her abuser, there could be a good reason for her accusation. Maybe the technology does exist. Or maybe he is using a different kind of device, which she does not yet understand. Or maybe the abuser has distorted her view of reality so much that she believes he can do impossible things, such as listen to her conversations through fillings in her teeth or read her mind.

Women who share children with their partners or former partners are in a particularly tough situation. Custody orders may conflict with orders of protection and provide avenues for stalking.

Professionals may feel tempted to create their own categories of "good" and "bad" victims. A "good" victim would be pretty, articulate, virtuous, feminine, friendly, weak, grateful, and obedient toward authorities. A victim who is upset, angry, intoxicated, unable to speak clear English, physically unattractive, or suspicious of authorities might seem less worthy of help. If the victim is an immigrant, LGBT, differently abled, or from a stigmatized racial minority group, professionals may find themselves drawing away, even if the victim truly needs their help. We must remember that those who may be least able to ask for help may be the people who need our help the most. Our work requires great patience and understanding, and an ability to truly listen to those who are suffering. All victims deserve our time, effort, and involvement.

12

Conclusion

Although they are not always effective, laws and social services exist to protect vulnerable people from their partners' physical violence. But physical violence is not the only danger that occurs in intimate relationships. We must make certain that abusers are not permitted to replace obvious physical violence with other forms of harmful coercive control.

Women have the right to their independence and freedom. When a woman is kept isolated and must use her time and energy to appease a controlling man, she not only suffers personally but is also unable to contribute fully to society and to her community. This is a loss for us all.

Men direct most of their violence toward other men. We cannot eliminate men's violence against women unless we directly face men's violence in general. Boys and men must learn ways to affirm themselves in their interactions that do not involve *power over* but rather *power together*. Parents, artists, social scientists, journalists, and educators all can help boys and men learn new, collaborative ways to express their masculinity. Cultural ideas of male and female roles must be broadened to make it easier for men to respect their partners' autonomy.

No one model of relating is right for all couples. Couples reach peace with different kinds of power arrangements, and within a couple these arrangements may change over time. Some people find contentment in relationships where they allow their partner to have more control, while others seek an ideal of mutual support, intimacy, and shared power. However, relationships become problematic when one person's fulfillment is *routinely sacrificed* in service of the other person. Threats, fear, and punishment do not belong in intimate relationships.

> **Relationships become problematic when one person's fulfillment is *routinely sacrificed* in service of the other's.**

Yes, it is important for us to help victims' efforts to escape from coercive control relationships and to support those abusers who want to change. But individual solutions alone cannot solve this broad social problem. Society must provide needed economic and educational resources for women to be able to support themselves and their children, and eventually achieve independence. We need to make sure the laws governing abusive couple relationships—and the way these laws are enforced—protect all victims of coercive entrapment and extreme forms of coercive control. We need to rewrite the laws on stalking and sexual coercion, to make sure they protect people who still live with their abusers. Living with or being married to an abuser does not mean a woman has consented to illegal assaults, stalking, and confinement within that relationship. The concept of coercive control should be discussed widely so people can recognize these relationships when they begin, and intervene.

Let's return to Mandy, discussed briefly in Chapter 1.

Mandy was 35 years old with two children and married to Tom, who increasingly controlled her, restricted her contact with her family, and made her feel trapped. Mandy had the support of a couple of long-term friends who called, e-mailed, and visited with her, even though Tom did not want her to see them often. Mostly, they helped Mandy feel good about herself. Mandy experienced an "a-ha moment" one morning when her 12-year-old asked her, "Mommy, why doesn't Daddy let you do anything?"

Mandy decided she had the right to determine her own fate, and she began to assert herself. She styled her hair the way she wanted and told Tom she was going to take a course online so she could finish her college degree and get a job. Tom tried to interfere, and Mandy decided she wanted to chart her own course.

Mandy contacted her local women's crisis agency, developed a safety plan, and told Tom the marriage was over. At first Tom tried to force Mandy to return by threatening to battle Mandy for custody of their children, and also by saying he would kill himself. Mandy's father, whom Tom respected, brought Tom to see a counselor who understood the concept of coercive control. The counselor helped Tom calm down and behave more reasonably, letting him know that continued threats might make him lose access to his children. Tom moved into a room in a friend's house, temporarily, so Mandy and the children could stay in their home. He signed up for a group for battering men and respected Mandy's wish that he contact her only when picking up the children on Saturdays, for his weekly visits. Time will tell whether Mandy and Tom will ever live together again—but she thinks it is not likely. Tom has resolved to change the way he relates to Mandy and all women so he can have healthier relationships in the future.

In this book, you have read stories of people who control their intimate partners by restricting their ability to make decisions about their own lives. Some of these decisions may seem small, but they add up. A woman should be able to decide for herself where she wants to go, with whom she wants to spend her time, and what she wants to eat and wear. If she has a partner, she will consider her partner's needs as she makes some of her decisions. But no person—including a spouse—should monopolize her time and thoughts. And she should not live in fear of punishment for putting her own desires and goals first, at least some of the time. She should not be expected to build her life entirely around her partner.

You have read about people from all walks of life who were victimized by coercive control. In these portrayals, maybe you have recognized yourself or others you know. You have seen what it means to be shackled by invisible chains, unable to make decisions, barred from spending time with others, and afraid of doing or saying the wrong thing.

Even though many people fear they will never find a way to break free from coercive control, happy endings are possible. Usually, victims need support, understanding, and material help from other people so they can emerge as survivors from these entrapping relationships. They need the love of friends and family, and the care of committed and knowledgeable professionals. The process of achieving freedom does not happen overnight, but it happens.

Resources

ESSENTIAL READINGS

Acker, S. E. (2013). *Unclenching our fists: Abusive men on the journey to non-violence*. Nashville, TN: Vanderbilt University Press.

This book shows how difficult it is for men who batter or emotionally abuse women to change their ways. But sometimes it is possible. The book provides in-depth interviews with culturally and economically diverse men who were once emotionally and/or physically violent with women and who overcame their violence through long, hard work in groups for battering men. After the interviews, Acker provides words of wisdom to women whose men say they are trying to overcome their battering.

Bancroft, L. (2002). *Why does he do that? Inside the minds of angry and controlling men*. New York: Putnam's Sons.

This book explains why angry and controlling men say and do the things they do. It describes their behaviors as a choice based on faulty thinking, rather than as impulsive outbursts.

Bancroft, L., & Patrissi, J. A. C. (2011). *Should I stay or should I go? A guide to knowing if your relationship can and should be saved.* New York: Berkley Books.

This book is designed to help women who are in relationships with abusive or destructive men reach a decision about the future of their relationships. It provides concrete advice and describes a program for reaching an informed decision. It helps readers separate the effects of their own actions and their partner's addictions, immaturity, mental illness, and abuse.

Stark, E. (2007). *Coercive control: How men entrap women in personal life.* New York: Oxford University Press.

This book describes and critiques the modern movement against intimate partner violence. It describes how many women who are battered by their partners are subject to treatment that resembles being held hostage more than it does assault by a stranger. The book advocates for changes in laws and attitudes regarding women victims of intimate partner violence, and tells the in-depth stories of three women who endured severe violence as well as near-constant control.

ORGANIZATIONS AND HELP LINES

In the United States

National Domestic Violence Hotline
www.thehotline.org

If you are in danger of domestic violence, call the National Domestic Violence Hotline, 1-800-799-SAFE (1-800-799-7233) or TTY 1-800-787-3224

National Sexual Violence Hotline
www.rainn.org/get-help/national-sexual-assualt-hotline

If you are in danger of sexual violence, call the National Sexual Violence Hotline, 1-800-656-HOPE (1-800-656-4673)

National Coalition Against Domestic Violence
www.ncadv.org

The NCADV is a coalition aimed at instituting legislative change to improve services and prevention for all communities victimized by domestic violence.

National Center on Domestic Violence, Trauma, and Mental Health
www.nationalcenterdvtraumamh.org

This organization aims to meet the mental health needs of survivors of domestic violence and their children across the lifespan. On their website they also have a list of United States domestic violence organizations, including those dedicated to helping victims from specific cultures.

National Indigenous Women's Resource Center
www.niwrc.org

The National Indigenous Women's Resource Center addresses domestic violence and safety for Indian women. The NIWRC seeks to enhance the capacity of American Indian and Alaska Native tribes, Native Hawaiians, and Tribal and Native Hawaiian organizations to respond to domestic violence.

National Network to End Domestic Violence
http://nnedv.org

NNEDV was founded by domestic violence survivors and works to make domestic violence a national priority, change the way communities respond to domestic violence, and strengthen efforts against intimate partner violence at every level of government.

Stalking Resource Center
www.victimsofcrime.org/our-programs/stalking-resource-center

This center provides resources, information, training, and support to the general public as well as professionals. It also provides links to local resources.

In Canada

Canada does not have a national center or organization; rather, each province has its own resources. For a list of resources by province, go to *www.casac.ca/content/anti-violence-centres*.

In England

If you are in danger of domestic violence, call 0808-2000-247.

Refuge
www.refuge.org.uk
Refuge provides shelter, advocacy, prevention, and culturally specific services to women and children affected by domestic violence.

Women's Aid
www.womensaid.org.uk
Women's Aid helps women and children throughout the United Kingdom and supports domestic and sexual violence services.

In Ireland

If you are in danger of domestic violence, call 1800-341-900.

Women's Aid Ireland
www.womensaid.ie

In Scotland

If you are in danger of domestic violence, call 0800-027-1234.

Scottish Women's Aid
www.scottishwomensaid.org.uk
The Scottish Women's Aid organization has resources pertaining directly to coercive control, in addition to intimate partner violence.

In Australia

If you are in danger of domestic violence, call 1-800-RESPECT (1-800-737-732).

National Sexual Assault, Family and Domestic Violence Counseling Line
www.1800respect.org.au
The website also has online counseling available 24 hours.

Women's Services Network
http://wesnet.org.au
WESNET is a national advocacy organization working on behalf of women and children who are experiencing or have experienced domestic or family violence.

In New Zealand

If you are in danger of domestic violence, call 0800-REFUGE or 0800-733-843.

Women's Refuge New Zealand
https://womensrefuge.org.nz
Women's Refuge is an organization for women and children dedicated to preventing and stopping family violence in New Zealand.

Speak Out Loud
http://speakoutloud.net
Speak Out Loud is a website dedicated to exploring coercive control. Its creator, Clare Murphy, PhD, is both a survivor of coercive control and a scholar of it. She offers blog posts on various aspects of coercive control relationships.

In India

For a list of domestic violence resources in India by region, go to *www.bellbajao.org/home/resources*.

References

1. Stark, E. (2007). *Coercive control: How men entrap women in personal life.* New York: Oxford University Press.

2. Johnson, M. P. (2008). *A typology of domestic violence: Intimate terrorism, violent resistance, and situational couple violence.* Boston: Northeastern University Press.

3. Hardesty, J. L., & Chung, G. H. (2006). Intimate partner violence, parental divorce, and child custody: Directions for intervention and future research. *Family Relations, 55,* 200–210.

4. Larrance, L. Y. (2006). Serving women who use force in their intimate heterosexual relationships: An extended view. *Violence Against Women, 12,* 622–640.

5. Wood, M., Barter, C., & Berridge, D. (2011). *'Standing on my own two feet': Disadvantaged teenagers, intimate partner violence and coercive control.* London: National Society for the Prevention of Cruelty to Children.

6. Levy-Peck, J. (2011). Sexual assault and coercion in teen relationships. Retrieved from *www.wcsap.org/sites/www.wcsap.org/files/uploads/webinars/Sexual%20Coercion%20in%20Teen%20Relationships/slides.pdf.*

7. Spitzberg, B. H., & Cupach, W. R. (2007). The state of the art of stalking: Taking stock of the emerging literature. *Aggression and Violent Behavior, 12,* 64–86.

8. Dunn, J. (2002). *Courting disaster: Intimate stalking, culture, and criminal justice.* New Brunswick, NJ: Aldine Transaction.

Index

Acknowledgments

My first offer of thanks and a deep bow must be to Evan Stark, PhD, whose groundbreaking 2007 book, *Coercive Control: The Entrapment of Women in Personal Life*, helped me understand violence against women in an entirely new way. Extremely supportive of this project, Evan generously commented on parts of an early draft of my book. Others who have provided descriptions of coercive control—sometimes with another name—include (in alphabetical order) David Adams, Lundy Bancroft, Connie Beck, Mary Ann Dutton, Patricia Evans, Anne Flitcraft, Lisa A. Goodman, Ann Jones, Michael P. Johnson, Del Martin, Beth E. Richie, and Susan Schechter. I'm sure I've missed someone, and for that I am deeply sorry. I salute these authors and the activists and survivors who work every day to reduce violence and achieve freedom for all the earth's people.

I thank those who read and shared their perceptions, encouragement, and critiques of versions of the manuscript and also shared their areas of expertise. This book has become much better with your help. In alphabetical order: Sara Elinoff Acker, Linda Baker, Genny Beemyn, Deb Bix, Kathy Conlon, Dawn DiStefano, Yolanda Fontanil, Ilana Gerjuoy, Kim Gerould, Magdalena

Gomez, Rachel Hare-Mustin, Karen Levine, Jay Loubris, Jenny Mason, Metta McGarvey, Cathy McSwain, Penni Micca, Kimber Nicoletti, Janine Roberts, Naomi Rosenblatt, and Robert Schmid.

I thank those friends, workshop participants, former clients, and others I've met along the way who have entrusted me with their stories. I hope I have done them justice. I apologize for any mistakes, oversights, or clumsiness in this book.

Many thanks to the team at The Guilford Press, most especially Chris Benton, Judith Grauman, and Kitty Moore, who believed in this project and have supported it from our first conversations.

A special thank you goes to those who helped me rise up and become myself again, especially: Sage Freechild, Ilana Gerjuoy, Lisa Lippiello, and Marian MacDonald. Thank you to the University of Massachusetts and Town of Amherst Police Departments and to Safe Passages in Northampton, Massachusetts, and the Center for Women and Community, Amherst, Massachusetts.

I became a writer and a feminist largely because my mother, Muriel Fox, showed me the way. I treasure her continued personal and professional support. Thanks, Mommy.

And to *mi gente* and *mishpucha*, my dear community of friends and family on several continents, who have supported me through good and bad times—you know who you are. I am so blessed! To Jay Loubris, who heard me cry and makes me laugh. And to Karen, Kim, Linda, and Wendy, hoping we can continue to count on each other, always.

Biggest hugs to my three spectacular children, Ana Lua, Marlena, and Gabriel Aronson Fontes. Each of you read and provided insightful suggestions on a draft of this book. Thank you for the inspiration, optimism, and happiness you give me each day. I yearn to see you and all the world's young people bask in kind and loving relationships.

I launch this book into the world hoping it will help people live and love, free from domination.

About the Author

Lisa Aronson Fontes, PhD, has a doctorate in counseling psychology and has worked in the areas of child abuse, violence against women, and challenging family issues for over 25 years. A professor, researcher, and popular conference speaker, she teaches at the University of Massachusetts Amherst. She survived a relationship that included coercive control and stalking. Her website is *www.lisafontes.com*.

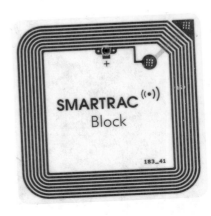